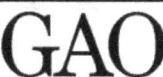

I0426153

February 2012

MEDICAL DEVICES

FDA Has Met Most Performance Goals but Device Reviews Are Taking Longer

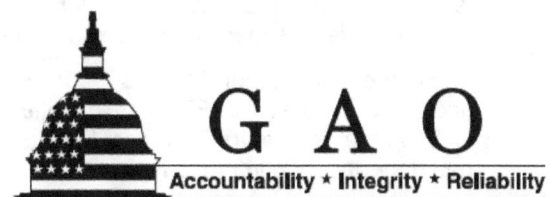

GAO
Accountability ★ Integrity ★ Reliability

GAO-12-418

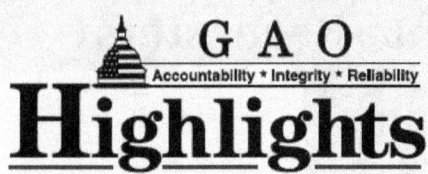

Highlights

Highlights of GAO-12-418, a report to congressional requesters

MEDICAL DEVICES

FDA Has Met Most Performance Goals but Device Reviews Are Taking Longer

Why GAO Did This Study

The Food and Drug Administration (FDA) within the Department of Health and Human Services (HHS) is responsible for overseeing the safety and effectiveness of medical devices sold in the United States. New devices are generally subject to FDA review via the 510(k) process, which determines if a device is substantially equivalent to another legally marketed device, or the more stringent premarket approval (PMA) process, which requires evidence providing reasonable assurance that the device is safe and effective. The Medical Device User Fee and Modernization Act of 2002 (MDUFMA) authorized FDA to collect user fees from the medical device industry to support the process of reviewing device submissions. FDA also committed to performance goals that include time frames within which FDA is to take action on a proportion of medical device submissions. MDUFMA was reauthorized in 2007.

Questions have been raised as to whether FDA is sufficiently meeting the performance goals and whether devices are reaching the market in a timely manner. In preparation for reauthorization, GAO was asked to (1) examine trends in FDA's 510(k) review performance from fiscal years (FY) 2003-2010, (2) examine trends in FDA's PMA review performance from FYs 2003-2010, and (3) describe stakeholder issues with FDA's review processes and steps FDA is taking that may address these issues. To do this work, GAO examined FDA medical device review data, reviewed FDA user fee data, interviewed FDA staff regarding the medical device review process and FDA data, and interviewed three industry groups and four consumer advocacy groups.

View GAO-12-418. For more information, contact Marcia Crosse at (202) 512-7114 or crossem@gao.gov.

What GAO Found

Even though FDA met all medical device performance goals for 510(k)s, the elapsed time from submission to final decision has increased substantially in recent years. This time to final decision includes the days FDA spends reviewing a submission as well as the days FDA spends waiting for a device sponsor to submit additional information in response to a request by the agency. FDA review time excludes this waiting time, and FDA review time alone is used to determine whether the agency met its performance goals. Each fiscal year since FY 2005 (the first year that 510(k) performance goals were in place), FDA has reviewed over 90 percent of 510(k) submissions within 90 days, thus meeting the first of two 510(k) performance goals. FDA also met the second goal for all 3 fiscal years it was in place by reviewing at least 98 percent of 510(k) submissions within 150 days. Although FDA has not yet completed reviewing all of the FY 2011 submissions, the agency was exceeding both of these performance goals for those submissions on which it had taken action. Although FDA review time decreased slightly from FY 2003 through FY 2010, the time that elapsed before FDA's final decision increased substantially. Specifically, from FY 2005 through FY 2010, the average time to final decision for 510(k)s increased 61 percent, from 100 days to 161 days.

FDA was inconsistent in meeting performance goals for PMA submissions. FDA designates PMAs as either original or expedited; those that FDA considers eligible for expedited review are devices intended to (a) treat or diagnose life-threatening or irreversibly debilitating conditions and (b) address an unmet medical need. While FDA met the performance goals for original PMA submissions for 4 out of 7 years the goals were in place, it met those goals for expedited PMA submissions only twice out of 7 years. FDA review time and time to final decision for both types of PMAs were highly variable but generally increased in recent years. For example, the average time to final decision for original PMAs increased from 462 days for FY 2003 to 627 days for FY 2008 (the most recent year for which complete data are available).

The three industry groups and four consumer advocacy groups GAO interviewed noted a number of issues related to FDA's review of medical device submissions. The four issues most commonly raised by stakeholders included (1) insufficient communication between FDA and stakeholders throughout the review process, (2) a lack of predictability and consistency in reviews, (3) an increase in time to final decision, and (4) inadequate assurance of the safety and effectiveness of approved or cleared devices. FDA is taking steps—including issuing new guidance documents, enhancing reviewer training, and developing an electronic system for reporting adverse events—that may address many of these issues. It is important for the agency to monitor the impact of those steps in ensuring that safe and effective medical devices are reaching the market in a timely manner.

In commenting on a draft of this report, HHS generally agreed with GAO's findings and noted that FDA has identified some of the same performance trends in its annual reports to Congress. HHS also called attention to the activities FDA has undertaken to improve the medical device review process.

Contents

Figures

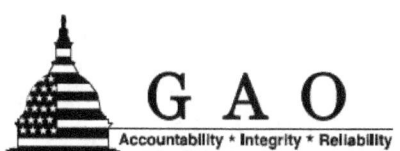

United States Government Accountability Office
Washington, DC 20548

February 29, 2012

The Honorable Richard Burr
Ranking Member
Subcommittee on Children and Families
Committee on Health, Education, Labor, and Pensions
United States Senate

The Honorable Tom Coburn
Ranking Member
Permanent Subcommittee on Investigations
Committee on Homeland Security and Governmental Affairs
United States Senate

The Food and Drug Administration (FDA) within the Department of Health and Human Services (HHS) is responsible for overseeing the safety and effectiveness of medical devices sold in the United States.[1] Congress passed the Medical Device User Fee and Modernization Act of 2002 (MDUFMA) to provide additional resources for FDA to support the process of reviewing medical device applications.[2] MDUFMA authorized FDA to collect user fees from the medical device industry to supplement its annual appropriation for salaries and expenses for fiscal years (FY) 2003 through 2007.[3] The medical device user fee program was reauthorized in 2007 as part of the Food and Drug Administration Amendments Act (FDAAA); the reauthorization was called the Medical Device User Fee Amendments of 2007 (MDUFA) and authorizes FDA to collect user fees for FYs 2008 through 2012.[4] FDA's authority to collect user fees for medical devices expires on October 1, 2012, and the

---

[1]Medical devices include instruments, apparatuses, machines, and implants that are intended for use to diagnose, cure, treat, or prevent disease, or to affect the structure or any function of the body. See 21 U.S.C. § 321(h). These devices range from simple tools such as bandages and surgical clamps to complicated devices such as pacemakers.

[2]See Pub. L. No. 107-250, § 102(a), 116 Stat. 1588, 1589-1600 (2002) (codified as amended at 21 U.S.C. §§ 379i and 379j).

[3]A user fee is a fee assessed for goods and services provided by the federal government. FDA collected one type of user fee—application fees—under MDUFMA.

[4]FDA collects three types of user fees under MDUFA: application fees, annual establishment registration fees, and annual fees for periodic reports regarding Class III devices.

medical device user fee program will need to be reauthorized for FDA to continue to collect user fees. Medical device user fee amounts have become a larger proportion of FDA's funding for medical device review processes, rising from 10.6 percent of costs in FY 2003—the first year FDA collected medical device user fees—to 19.5 percent of costs in FY 2010, the most recent year for which data are available. In FY 2010, MDUFA user fees collected by FDA—including application, establishment, and product fees—totaled nearly $67 million, including over $29 million in application fees.[5] Application fees are collected for a variety of medical device submission types, including premarket notifications (510(k)s) and premarket approvals (PMAs).[6]

Under each authorization of the medical device user fee program, FDA committed to performance goals related to the review of medical device submissions.[7] The performance goals include specific time frames within which FDA is to take action on submissions.[8] These performance goals, as well as user fee amounts, are negotiated between FDA and industry stakeholders and submitted to congressional committees prior to each reauthorization. Questions have been raised about whether FDA is sufficiently meeting the user fee performance goals and whether medical devices are reaching the market in a timely manner. A number of congressional committees have recently held hearings during which the

---

[5]For the remainder of this report, we use the term "user fees" to refer to user fees submitted with device applications such as premarket approvals (PMA), premarket notifications (510(k)), and various types of PMA supplements.

[6]The PMA review process is more stringent than the 510(k) review process and is generally used for higher risk devices. As part of a PMA submission, the manufacturer is required to supply evidence providing reasonable assurance that the device is safe and effective. Under the 510(k) process, FDA determines whether the device is substantially equivalent to a legally marketed device. FDA also reviews several other types of medical device submissions that are outside the scope of our work. PMAs and 510(k)s make up the majority of device submissions received by FDA. For example, our analysis of PMAs and 510(k)s included 88.6 percent of all device submissions to FDA in FY 2010.

[7]See Pub. L. No. 110-85, § 201(c), 121 Stat. 823, 842-43 (2007). The performance goals are identified in letters sent by the Secretary of Health and Human Services to the Chairman of the Senate Committee on Health, Education, Labor, and Pensions and the Chairman of the House Committee on Energy and Commerce and are published on FDA's website. Each fiscal year, FDA is required to submit a report on its progress in achieving those goals and future plans for meeting them. See 21 U.S.C. § 379j-1(a).

[8]FDA does not have to approve a PMA or clear a 510(k) for it to be considered acted upon. There are a number of decisions in addition to an approval or clearance decision that can end FDA's review.

medical device industry questioned FDA's timeliness, while other stakeholders questioned FDA's ability to ensure safety and effectiveness.

In preparation for the reauthorization of the medical device user fee program, you requested that we examine FDA's medical device review process. In this report, we (1) examine trends in FDA's 510(k) medical device review performance for FYs 2003 through 2010, (2) examine trends in FDA's PMA medical device review performance for FYs 2003 through 2010, and (3) describe the issues stakeholders have raised about the medical device review processes and steps FDA is taking that may address these issues. We provide additional details on FDA's medical device review performance in appendix I. You also asked us to provide information on the number of full-time equivalent (FTE) staff involved in the medical device review process; this information is provided in appendix II.

To determine the trends in FDA's medical device review performance for 510(k)s and PMAs for FYs 2003 through 2010, we examined data obtained from FDA on the review process for all 510(k)s and PMAs submitted to FDA in those years.[9] To provide context for FDA's performance prior to enactment of the user fee acts, we also analyzed review data for all 510(k)s and PMAs submitted for FYs 2000 through 2002. Additionally, we reviewed data on FY 2011 submissions in order to provide preliminary performance results for that year.[10] Our analyses focused on the proportion of medical device submissions in each fiscal year for which FDA met or did not meet the applicable performance goal(s); the total time from the date of submission to the date a final decision was made—including both the time FDA spent reviewing a submission and any time the sponsor took to respond to questions or requests for additional information from FDA; the FDA review time (i.e., the time counted toward user fee performance goals, which does not include any time the sponsor took to respond to any questions from FDA);

---

[9] We defined a cohort to be complete if fewer than 10 percent of submissions from that cohort were still under review at the time we received FDA's data.

[10] The data for FY 2011 are preliminary because the agency had only completed its review for 61 percent of 510(k) submissions and 51 percent of PMA submissions at the time we received FDA's data. As a result, it was too soon to tell what the final results for this cohort would be. For example, it is possible that some of the reviews taking the most time were among those not completed when we received FDA's data.

and the average number of review cycles prior to approval.[11] We also reviewed publicly available FDA user fee data for FY 2003 through 2010 and interviewed FDA staff regarding the medical device review process and the data we received from FDA.

To describe the issues stakeholders have raised about the device review processes and what steps FDA is taking that may address these issues, we reviewed congressional testimony and interviewed three industry groups and four consumer advocacy groups.[12] All of these groups have participated in at least half of the meetings held by FDA to discuss the reauthorization of the user fee program. Furthermore, the industry groups we interviewed represent a mixture of large and small medical device manufacturers and cover a significant portion of the device market. We performed content analyses of the interviews to determine the most pressing issues based on how often each issue was raised.[13]

We conducted this performance audit from October 2011 through February 2012 in accordance with generally accepted government auditing standards. Those standards require that we plan and perform the audit to obtain sufficient, appropriate evidence to provide a reasonable basis for our findings and conclusions based on our audit objectives. We believe that the evidence obtained provides a reasonable basis for our findings and conclusions based on our audit objectives.

Background

Medical devices are reviewed primarily by FDA's Center for Devices and Radiological Health (CDRH), with a smaller proportion reviewed by the Center for Biologics Evaluation and Research (CBER). FDA classifies each device type into one of three classes—class I, II, or III—based on the level of risk it poses and the controls necessary to reasonably ensure

---

[11]The first review cycle begins when a sponsor makes a submission to FDA and ends when FDA either makes a decision or contacts the sponsor in writing to request additional information. A new review cycle begins when the sponsor sends a response back to FDA.

[12]When we refer to consumer advocacy groups, we are referring to groups that advocate on behalf of consumers and patients.

[13]It was beyond the scope of our review to describe all issues raised by stakeholders. Such issues—including barriers to innovation in the medical device industry or the need for increased resources at FDA—have been extensively covered in other reports, forums, and hearings.

its safety and effectiveness.[14] Class I includes devices with the lowest risk (e.g., tongue depressors, reading glasses, forceps), while class III includes devices with the highest risk (e.g., breast implants, coronary stents). Almost all class I devices and some class II devices (e.g., mercury thermometers, certain adjustable hospital beds) are exempt from premarket notification requirements. Most class III device types are required to obtain FDA approval through the PMA process, the most stringent of FDA's medical device review processes.[15] The remaining device types are required to obtain FDA clearance or approval through either the 510(k) or PMA processes.[16]

If eligible, a 510(k) is filed when a manufacturer seeks a determination that a new device is substantially equivalent to a legally marketed device known as a predicate device.[17] In order to be deemed substantially equivalent (i.e., cleared by FDA for marketing), a new device must have the same technological characteristics and intended use as the predicate device, or have the same intended use and different technological characteristics but still be demonstrated to be as safe and effective as the predicate device without raising new questions of safety and effectiveness. Most device submissions filed each year are 510(k)s. For

---

[14]See 21 U.S.C. § 360c(a)(1); 21 C.F.R. pt. 860.

[15]Some class III device types on the market before the enactment of the Medical Device Amendments of 1976 and those determined to be substantially equivalent to them do not currently require PMA approval for marketing. FDA has been taking steps to address these device types; once this process is completed, all class III devices will be required to go through the PMA review process. For additional information, see GAO, *Medical Devices: FDA's Premarket Review and Postmarket Safety Efforts*, GAO-11-556T (Washington, D.C.: Apr. 13, 2011).

[16]A small percentage of devices enter the market by other means, such as through the humanitarian device exemption process that authorizes FDA to exempt certain medical devices from the premarket review requirement to demonstrate effectiveness in order to provide an incentive for the development of devices that treat or diagnose rare diseases or conditions. See 21 U.S.C. § 360j(m); 21 C.F.R. pt. 814, subpt. H.

[17]A legally marketed device to which a new device may be compared for a determination regarding substantial equivalence is a device that was legally marketed prior to 1976, a device that has been reclassified from class III to class II or I, or a device that has been found to be substantially equivalent through the 510(k) process. See 21 C.F.R. § 807.92(a)(3).

example, of the more than 13,600 device submissions received by FDA in FYs 2008 through 2010, 88 percent were 510(k)s.[18]

The medical device performance goals were phased in during the period covered by MDUFMA (the FYs 2003 through 2007 cohorts) and were updated for MDUFA.[19] Under MDUFA, FDA's goal is to complete the review process for 90 percent of the 510(k)s in a cohort within 90 days of submission (known as the Tier 1 goal) and to complete the review process for 98 percent of the cohort within 150 days (the Tier 2 goal).[20] (See table 1 for the 510(k) performance goals for the FYs 2003 through 2011 cohorts). FDA may take any of the following actions on a 510(k) after completing its review:

- issue an order declaring the device substantially equivalent;

- issue an order declaring the device not substantially equivalent; or

- advise the submitter that the 510(k) is not required (i.e., the product is not regulated as a device or the device is exempt from premarket notification requirements).

---

[18]See Department of Health and Human Services, Food and Drug Administration, *Quarterly Update on Medical Device Performance Goals* (Silver Spring, Md.: July 26, 2011).

[19]A cohort is comprised of all the submissions of a certain type filed in the same fiscal year. For example, all 510(k)s received by FDA from October 1, 2010, to September 30, 2011, make up the 510(k) review cohort for FY 2011.

[20]Tier 1 and Tier 2 designations refer to the length of time allotted (90 days and 150 days, respectively) for FDA to complete its review of 510(k) submissions. If FDA completed its review of a submission in 90 days or less, it met the time frame for both the Tier 1 and Tier 2 goals. If the review was completed in more than 90 days but not more than 150 days, only the time frame for the Tier 2 goal was met. If the review took longer than 150 days, the time frame for neither goal was met. FDA did not designate 510(k) performance goals as either Tier 1 or Tier 2 prior to FY 2008. We have aligned the performance goals in place prior to FY 2008 with the Tier 1 goals for FYs 2008-2011 based on sharing the same 90-day time frame. This placement illustrates the increase in the goal percentage over time. We defined a 510(k) cohort to be complete if fewer than 10 percent of submissions from that cohort were still under review at the time we received FDA's data, which cover reviews by CDRH through October 26, 2011, and reviews by CBER through December 23, 2011. Using this definition, FY 2011 was the only 510(k) cohort that was incomplete.

Each of these actions ends the review process for a submission.[21] A sponsor's withdrawal of a submission also ends the review process.

Table 1: FDA's 510(k) Performance Goals, FYs 2003-2011

Fiscal year cohort	Period covered by MDUFMA					Period covered by MDUFA[a]			
	2003	2004	2005	2006	2007	2008	2009	2010	2011
Tier 1 goal percentage[b]	—	—	75[c]	75[c]	80[c]	90	90	90	90
Tier 2 goal percentage[d]	—	—	—	—	—	98	98	98	98

Source: GAO analysis of FDA data.

Notes: A review cohort includes all the medical device submissions relating to a particular performance goal that were submitted in a given fiscal year. For example, all 510(k)s received by FDA from October 1, 2010, to September 30, 2011, make up the 510(k) review cohort for FY 2011.

There were no 510(k) performance goals prior to MDUFMA. Fiscal years for which there was no corresponding 510(k) performance goal are denoted with a dash (—).

[a]MDUFA performance goals cover the FYs 2008 through 2012 cohorts; we are showing only those cohorts we examined as part of our analysis.

[b]Percentage of 510(k) submissions to be completed by FDA within 90 days of submission.

[c]These were not designated as Tier 1 goals prior to FY 2008 because there were no Tier 2 goals for those cohorts. We have aligned them with the Tier 1 goals for FYs 2008 through 2011 because they are based on the same 90-day time frame and this placement illustrates the gradual increase in the goal percentage over time.

[d]Percentage of 510(k) submissions to be completed by FDA within 150 days of submission.

Alternatively, FDA may "stop the clock" on a 510(k) review by sending a letter asking the sponsor to submit additional information (known as an AI letter). This completes a review cycle but does not end the review process. The clock will resume (and a new review cycle will begin) when FDA receives a response from the sponsor. As a result, FDA may meet its 510(k) performance goals even if the time to final decision (FDA review time plus time spent waiting for the sponsor to respond to FDA's requests for additional information) is longer than the time frame allotted for the performance goal. For example, a sponsor might have submitted a 510(k) on March 1, 2009, to start the review process. If FDA sent an AI letter on April 1, 2009 (after 31 days on the clock), the sponsor provided a response on June 1, 2009 (after an additional 61 days off the clock), and FDA issued a final decision on June 11, 2009 (10 more days on the

---

[21]When calculating whether FDA met the performance goal for a 510(k) cohort, FDA and industry have agreed to include only those submissions receiving a substantially equivalent or not substantially equivalent decision. For our analysis, we included all 510(k)s that had received a final decision, regardless of the decision received, in order to provide a broader look at FDA's review performance.

clock), then the FDA review time counted toward the MDUFA performance goals would be 41 days (FDA's on-the-clock time). FDA would have met both the Tier 1 (90 day) and Tier 2 (150 day) time frames for that device even though the total number of calendar days (on- and off-the-clock) from beginning the review to a final decision was 102 days. (See table 2 for a comparison of FDA review time and time to final decision.) FDA tracks the time to final decision and reports on it in the agency's annual reports to Congress on the medical device user fee program.[22]

Table 2: GAO Definitions of FDA Review Time and Time to Final Decision

Term	Definition
FDA review time	The time used to determine whether FDA met the medical device user fee performance goals. Determined by counting the on-the-clock time that FDA spends reviewing a submission during all review cycles and does not include any time that FDA spends between review cycles waiting for the sponsor to submit additional information.
Time to final decision	The total elapsed time from the date of submission through the date of FDA's final decision. Determined by adding on-the-clock time (FDA review time) for all review cycles and any off-the-clock time that FDA spends between review cycles waiting for the sponsor to submit additional information.

Source: GAO.

A PMA is filed when a device is not substantially equivalent to a predicate device or has been classified as a class III PMA device (when the risks associated with the device are considerable). The PMA review process is the most stringent type of medical device review process required by FDA, and user fees are much higher for PMAs than for 510(k)s.[23] PMAs are designated as either original or expedited.[24] FDA considers a device eligible for expedited review if it is intended to (a) treat or diagnose a life-threatening or irreversibly debilitating disease or condition and

---

[22]In its July 2011 analysis of 510(k) submissions, FDA concluded that reviewers asked for additional information from sponsors—thus stopping the clock on FDA's review time while the total time to reach a final decision continued to elapse—mainly due to problems with the quality of the submission. See U.S. Department of Health and Human Services, Food and Drug Administration, *Analysis of Premarket Review Times Under the 510(k) Program* (Silver Spring, Md.: July 2011).

[23]For example, for FY 2012 the standard PMA application fee is $220,050 while the 510(k) fee is $4,049.

[24]In its annual performance reports, FDA refers to these two types as original PMAs and expedited original PMAs.

(b) address an unmet medical need.[25] FDA assesses all medical device submissions to determine which are appropriate for expedited review, regardless of whether a company has identified its device as a potential candidate for this program.

To meet the MDUFA goals, FDA must complete its review of 60 percent of the original PMAs in a cohort within 180 days of submission (Tier 1) and 90 percent within 295 days (Tier 2). For expedited PMAs, 50 percent of a cohort must be completed within 180 days (Tier 1) and 90 percent within 280 days (Tier 2). (See table 3 for the PMA performance goals for the FYs 2003 through 2011 cohorts.) The various actions FDA may take during its review of a PMA are the following:

- approval order;

- approvable letter;

- major deficiency letter;

- not approvable letter; and

- denial order.[26]

---

[25]See 21 U.S.C. § 360e(d)(5). Unmet medical need is demonstrated by meeting one of the following criteria: the device represents a breakthrough technology that provides a clinically meaningful advantage over existing technology; no approved alternative treatment or means of diagnosis exists; the device offers significant, clinically meaningful advantages over existing approved alternative treatments; or the availability of the device is in the best interest of patients.

[26]An approval order informs the applicant that the PMA has been approved. An approvable letter is sent to inform the applicant that there needs to be resolution of minor deficiencies or completion of an FDA inspection. A major deficiency letter informs the applicant that the PMA lacks significant information necessary for the agency to complete its review and requests the applicant amend the submission to provide the necessary information. A not approvable letter informs the applicant that the submission cannot be approved at that time because of significant deficiencies; describes the deficiencies; and, where practical, describes the measures required to make the submission approvable. Generally, before FDA issues a not approvable letter, it will first issue a major deficiency letter to provide the applicant with an opportunity to address its concerns. A denial order notifies the applicant that the PMA is not approved and informs the applicant of its deficiencies.

The major deficiency letter is the only one of these actions that does not end the review process for purposes of determining whether FDA met the MDUFA performance goal time frame for a given submission. As with the AI letter in a 510(k) review, FDA can stop the clock during the PMA review process by sending a major deficiency letter (ending a review cycle) and resume it later upon receiving a response from the manufacturer. In contrast, taking one of the other four actions permanently stops the clock, meaning any further review that occurs is excluded from the calculation of FDA review time. In addition, the approval order and denial order are also considered final decisions and end FDA's review of a PMA completely. A sponsor's withdrawal of a submission also ends the review process.

Table 3: FDA's PMA Performance Goals, FYs 2003-2011

Fiscal year cohort	Period covered by MDUFMA					Period covered by MDUFA[a]			
	2003	2004	2005[b]	2006[b]	2007[b]	2008	2009	2010	2011
Original PMA Tier 1 goal percentage[c]	—	—	—	—	50	60	60	60	60
Original PMA Tier 2 goal percentage[d]	—	—	—	80	90	90	90	90	90
Expedited PMA Tier 1 goal percentage[e]	—	—	—	—	—	50	50	50	50
Expedited PMA Tier 2 goal percentage[f]	—	—	70	80	90	90	90	90	90

Source: GAO analysis of FDA data.

Notes: A review cohort includes all the medical device submissions relating to a particular performance goal that were submitted in a given fiscal year. For example, all PMAs received by FDA from October 1, 2010, to September 30, 2011, make up the PMA review cohort for FY 2011.

There were no performance goals prior to MDUFMA. Fiscal years for which there was no corresponding PMA performance goal are denoted with a dash (—).

[a]MDUFA performance goals cover the FYs 2008 through 2012 cohorts; we are showing only those cohorts we examined as part of our analysis.

[b]PMA performance goals were not designated as Tier 1 or Tier 2 until FY 2008. We have aligned the performance goals in place prior to FY 2008 with the Tier 1 or Tier 2 goals for FYs 2008 through 2011 based on sharing the same or similar goal time frames. This placement illustrates the increase in the goal percentage over time.

[c]Percentage of original PMAs to be completed by FDA within 180 days of submission.

[d]Percentage of original PMAs to be completed by FDA within 320 days (for FYs 2006 through 2007) or 295 days (FYs 2008 through 2011) of submission.

[e]Percentage of expedited PMAs to be completed by FDA within 180 days of submission.

[f]Percentage of expedited PMAs to be completed by FDA within 300 days (for FYs 2005 through 2007) or 280 days (FYs 2008 through 2011) of submission.

FDA's review of medical device submissions has been discussed in recent congressional hearings, meetings between FDA and stakeholders about the medical device user fee program reauthorization, and published reports. In addition, in August 2010, FDA released reports which described the results of two internal assessments conducted by FDA of its medical device review programs.[27] In January 2011, FDA released a plan of action that included 25 steps FDA intends to take to address the issues identified in these assessments.[28]

FDA Met All Performance Goals for 510(k)s but the Time to Final Decision Has Increased Substantially in Recent Years

For FYs 2003 through 2010, FDA met all Tier 1 and Tier 2 performance goals for 510(k)s. In addition, FDA review time for 510(k)s decreased slightly during this period, but time to final decision increased substantially. The average number of review cycles and FDA's requests for additional information for 510(k) submissions also increased during this period.

[27]In September 2009, FDA convened an internal 510(k) working group to conduct a comprehensive assessment of the 510(k) process. This assessment resulted in the publication of a preliminary report in August 2010, which was intended to communicate preliminary findings and recommendations and actions FDA might take to address identified areas of concern. See U.S. Department of Health and Human Services, Food and Drug Administration, *510(k) Working Group: Preliminary Report and Recommendations* (Silver Spring, Md.: August 2010). Also in September 2009, FDA convened an internal task force on the utilization of science in regulatory decision making. This task force was responsible for reviewing how FDA uses science in its regulatory decision making for device reviews and making recommendations on how FDA can quickly incorporate new science—including evolving information, novel technologies, and new scientific methods—into its decision making, while maintaining as much predictability as practical. The task force released a preliminary report with its findings and recommendations in August 2010. See U.S. Department of Health and Human Services, Food and Drug Administration, *Task Force on the Utilization of Science in Regulatory Decision Making, Preliminary Report and Recommendations* (Silver Spring, Md.: August 2010).

[28]In January 2011, after reviewing public comments on the August 2010 reports, FDA issued a plan of action for implementing the recommendations in the reports. See U.S. Department of Health and Human Services, Food and Drug Administration, *Plan of Action for Implementation of 510(k) and Science Recommendations* (Silver Spring, Md.: January 2011). FDA began implementing these actions in March 2011 and the majority of the actions had been implemented or were underway at the time of our report. See U.S. Department of Health and Human Services, Food and Drug Administration, *CDRH Plan of Action for 510(k) and Science* (Silver Spring, Md.: October 2011).

FDA Met All Tier 1 and Tier 2 Performance Goals for 510(k)s from 2003 through 2010

FDA met all Tier 1 performance goals for the completed 510(k) cohorts that had Tier 1 goals in place.[29] The percentage of 510(k)s reviewed within 90 days (the current Tier 1 goal time frame) exceeded 90 percent for the FYs 2005 through 2010 cohorts (see fig. 1.) Although the 510(k) cohort for FY 2011 was still incomplete at the time we received FDA's data, FDA was exceeding the Tier 1 goal for those submissions on which it had taken action.[30] FDA's performance varied for 510(k) cohorts prior to the years that the Tier 1 goals were in place but was always below the current 90 percent goal.

---

[29]When calculating whether FDA met the performance goal for a 510(k) cohort, FDA and industry have agreed to include only those submissions receiving a substantially equivalent or not substantially equivalent decision. For our analysis, we included all 510(k)s that had received a final decision, regardless of the decision received, in order to provide a broader look at FDA's review performance.

[30]Approximately 39 percent of 510(k)s received in FY 2011 were still under review at the time we received FDA's data, which cover reviews by CDRH through October 26, 2011, and reviews by CBER through December 23, 2011. As a result, it was too soon to tell what the final results for this cohort would be. For example, the percentage of completed 510(k)s that met the 90-day performance goal time frame was 97.2 percent. However, the percentage of 510(k)s reviewed within 90 days for the FY 2011 cohort may increase or decrease as those reviews are completed.

Figure 1: Percentage of 510(k)s FDA Reviewed within 90 Days for the Fiscal Year 2000-2010 Cohorts

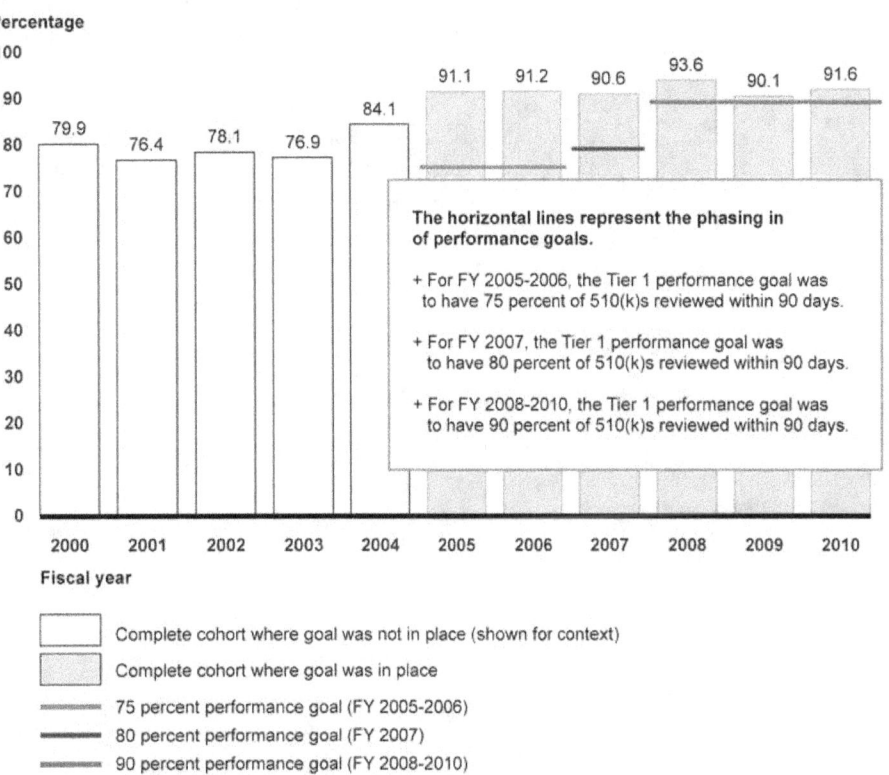

Source: GAO analysis of FDA data.

Note: Only 510(k)s that had received a final decision from FDA were included in this analysis. Tier 1 and Tier 2 designations refer to the length of time allotted (90 days and 150 days, respectively) for FDA to complete its review of 510(k) submissions. If FDA completed its review of a 510(k) submission in 90 days or less, it met the time frames for both the Tier 1 and Tier 2 goals. If the review was completed in more than 90 days but not more than 150 days, only the time frame for the Tier 2 goal was met. If the review took longer than 150 days, FDA did not meet the time frame for either goal. FDA did not designate 510(k) performance goals as either Tier 1 or Tier 2 prior to FY 2008. We have aligned the performance goals in place prior to FY 2008 with the Tier 1 goals for FYs 2008 through 2011 based on sharing the same 90-day time frame. This placement illustrates the increase in the goal percentage over time.

FDA met the Tier 2 goals for all three of the completed cohorts that had Tier 2 goals in place. Specifically, FDA met the goal of reviewing 98 percent of submissions within 150 days for the FYs 2008, 2009, and 2010 cohorts (see fig. 2.) Additionally, although the 510(k) cohort for FY 2011 was still incomplete at the time we received FDA's data, FDA was exceeding the Tier 2 goal for those submissions on which it had taken action.[31] FDA's performance for 510(k) cohorts prior to the years that the Tier 2 goals were in place was generally below the current 98 percent goal.

[31]Approximately 39 percent of 510(k)s received in FY 2011 were still under review at the time we received FDA's data, which cover reviews by CDRH through October 26, 2011, and reviews by CBER through December 23, 2011. As a result, it was too soon to tell what the final results for this cohort would be. For example, the percentage of completed 510(k)s that met the 150-day performance goal was 99.8 percent. However, the percentage of 510(k)s reviewed within 150 days for the FY 2011 cohort may increase or decrease as those reviews are completed.

Figure 2: Percentage of 510(k)s FDA Reviewed within 150 Days for the Fiscal Year 2000-2010 Cohorts

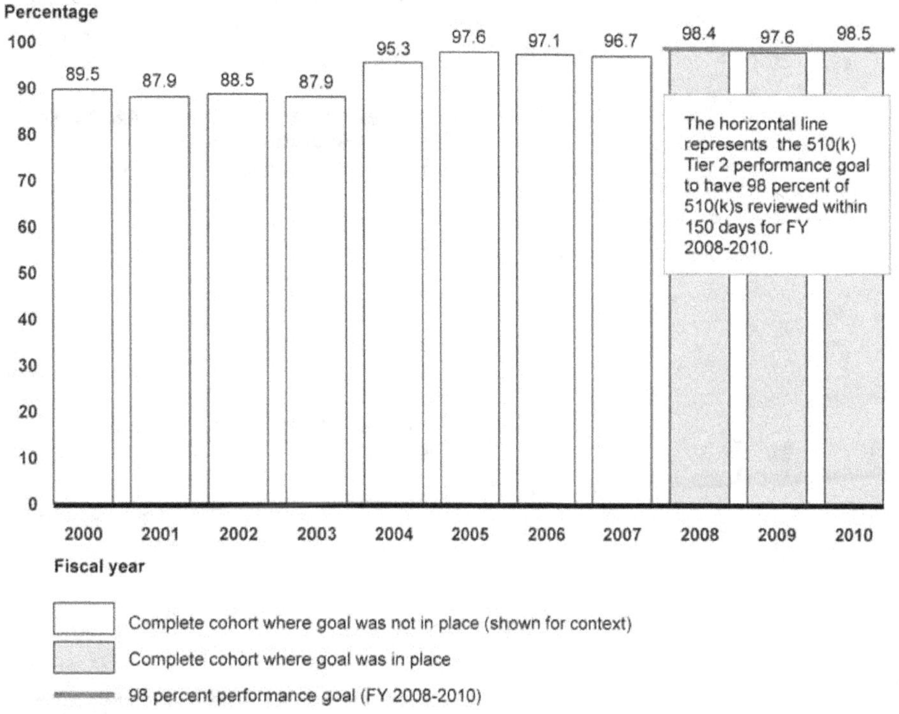

Percentage

2000	89.5
2001	87.9
2002	88.5
2003	87.9
2004	95.3
2005	97.6
2006	97.1
2007	96.7
2008	98.4
2009	97.6
2010	98.5

The horizontal line represents the 510(k) Tier 2 performance goal to have 98 percent of 510(k)s reviewed within 150 days for FY 2008-2010.

Fiscal year

☐ Complete cohort where goal was not in place (shown for context)

▨ Complete cohort where goal was in place

▬ 98 percent performance goal (FY 2008-2010)

Source: GAO analysis of FDA data.

Note: Only 510(k)s that had received a final decision from FDA were included in this analysis. For purposes of determining whether a goal was met, the percentage is rounded to the nearest whole number. Tier 1 and Tier 2 designations refer to the length of time allotted (90 days and 150 days, respectively) for FDA to complete its review of 510(k) submissions. If FDA completed its review of a submission in 90 days or less, it met the time frames for both the Tier 1 and Tier 2 goals. If the review was completed in more than 90 days but not more than 150 days, only the time frame for the Tier 2 goal was met. If the review took longer than 150 days, FDA did not meet the time frame for either goal. FDA did not designate 510(k) performance goals as either Tier 1 or Tier 2 prior to FY 2008.

FDA Review Time for 510(k)s Decreased Slightly from 2003 to 2010 but Time to Final Decision Increased Substantially

While the average FDA review time for 510(k) submissions decreased slightly from the FY 2003 cohort to the FY 2010 cohort, the time to final decision increased substantially. Specifically, the average number of days FDA spent on the clock reviewing a 510(k) varied somewhat but overall showed a small decrease from 75 days for the FY 2003 cohort to 71 days for the FY 2010 cohort (see fig. 3). However, when we added off-the-clock time (where FDA waited for the sponsor to provide additional information) to FDA's on-the-clock review time, the resulting time to final decision decreased slightly from the FY 2003 cohort to the FY 2005 cohort before increasing 61 percent—from 100 days to 161 days—from the FY 2005 cohort through the FY 2010 cohort. FDA officials told us that the only alternative to requesting additional information is for FDA to reject the submission. The officials stated that as a result of affording sponsors this opportunity to respond, the time to final decision is longer but the application has the opportunity to be approved.

Figure 3: Average FDA Review Time and Average Time to Final Decision for 510(k)s in the Fiscal Year 2000-2010 Cohorts

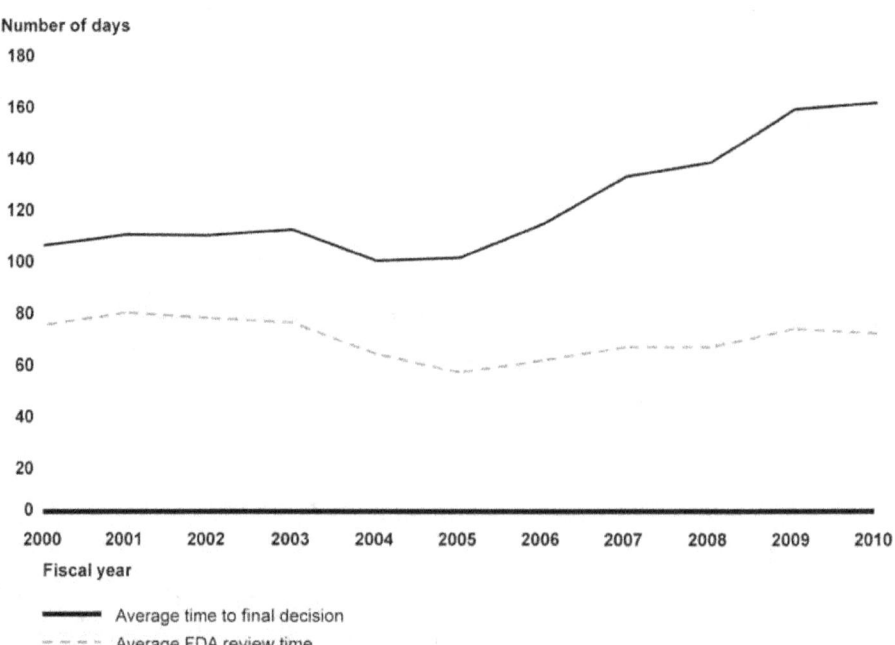

Source: GAO analysis of FDA data.

Note: Only 510(k)s that had received a final decision from FDA were included in this analysis. Average FDA review time refers to the time that FDA spends reviewing a submission and therefore excludes any time the sponsor may spend responding to FDA requests for additional information. Average time to final decision includes both the time FDA spends reviewing a submission and the time the sponsor may spend responding to any requests for additional information.

Additionally, although the 510(k) cohort for FY 2011 was still incomplete at the time we received FDA's data, the average FDA review time and time to final decision were lower in FY 2011 for those submissions on which it had taken action.[32]

Number of Review Cycles and Requests for Additional Information Increased for 510(k) Submissions from 2003 to 2010

The average number of review cycles per 510(k) increased substantially (39 percent) from FYs 2003 through 2010, rising from 1.47 cycles for the FY 2003 cohort to 2.04 cycles for the FY 2010 cohort (see fig. 4).

Figure 4: Average Number of Review Cycles Per 510(k) for the Fiscal Year 2000-2010 Cohorts

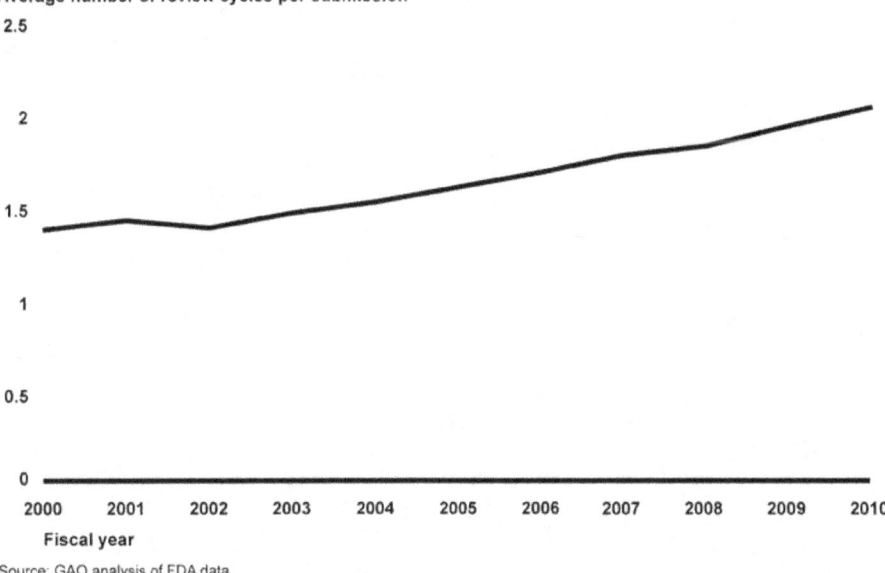

Source: GAO analysis of FDA data.

Note: Cycles that were currently in progress at the time we received FDA's data were included in this analysis.

---

[32]Approximately 39 percent of 510(k)s received in FY 2011 were still under review at the time we received FDA's data, which cover reviews by CDRH through October 26, 2011, and reviews by CBER through December 23, 2011. As a result, it was too soon to tell what the final results for this cohort would be. It is possible that some of the reviews taking the most time were among those not completed when we received FDA's data.

In addition, the percentage of 510(k)s receiving a first-cycle decision of substantially equivalent (i.e., cleared by FDA for marketing) decreased from 54 percent for the FY 2003 cohort to 20 percent for the FY 2010 cohort, while the percentage receiving first-cycle AI requests exhibited a corresponding increase. (See fig. 5.) The average number of 510(k) submissions per year remained generally steady during this period. Although the 510(k) cohort for FY 2011 was still incomplete at the time we received FDA's data, of the first-cycle reviews that had been completed, the percentage of submissions receiving a first-cycle decision of substantially equivalent was slightly higher than for the FY 2010 cohort (21.2 percent in FY 2011 compared with 20.0 percent in FY 2010).[33] In addition, the percentage receiving a first-cycle AI request was lower (68.2 percent for FY 2011 compared with 77.0 for FY 2010).[34]

---

[33]Approximately 39 percent of 510(k)s received in FY 2011 were still under review at the time we received FDA's data, which cover reviews by CDRH through October 26, 2011, and reviews by CBER through December 23, 2011. As a result, it was too soon to tell what the final results for this cohort would be. Therefore, the percentage of 510(k)s in the FY 2011 cohort receiving a first-cycle substantially equivalent decision may increase or decrease as those reviews are completed.

[34]Approximately 39 percent of 510(k)s received in FY 2011 were still under review at the time we received FDA's data, which cover reviews by CDRH through October 26, 2011, and reviews by CBER through December 23, 2011. As a result, it was too soon to tell what the final results for this cohort would be. Therefore, the percentage of 510(k)s in the FY 2011 cohort receiving a first-cycle AI letter may increase or decrease as those reviews are completed.

Figure 5: Percentage of 510(k) Submissions Receiving FDA First-Cycle Substantially Equivalent Decisions and First-Cycle Additional Information Requests for the Fiscal Year 2000-2010 Cohorts

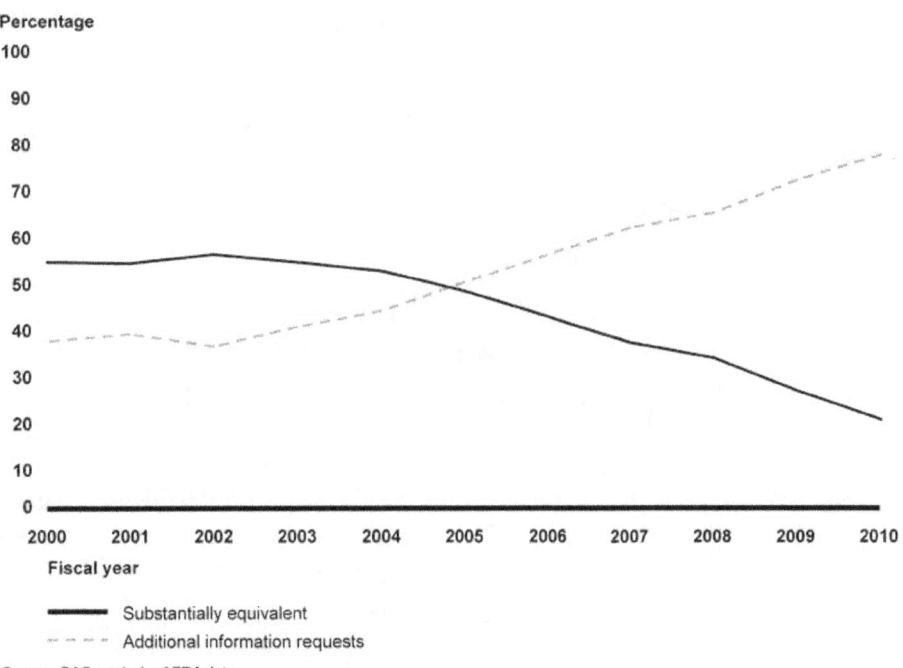

Source: GAO analysis of FDA data.

Notes: Only 510(k)s that had received a first-cycle decision from FDA were included in this analysis.

The percentages for each year do not add to 100 percent because there are other possible actions classified as first-cycle decisions (e.g., a sponsor's withdrawal of a submission).

The first review cycle starts when FDA receives a submission and ends when FDA either makes a decision regarding substantial equivalence or requests additional information from the sponsor, or the sponsor withdraws the submission. More than one cycle may occur before FDA reaches its final decision.

The percentage of 510(k)s that received a final decision of substantially equivalent also decreased in recent years—from a high of 87.9 percent for the FY 2005 cohort down to 75.1 percent for the FY 2010 cohort. The percentage of 510(k)s receiving a final decision of not substantially equivalent increased for each cohort from FYs 2003 through 2010, rising from just over 2.9 percent to 6.4 percent. (See fig. 6.)

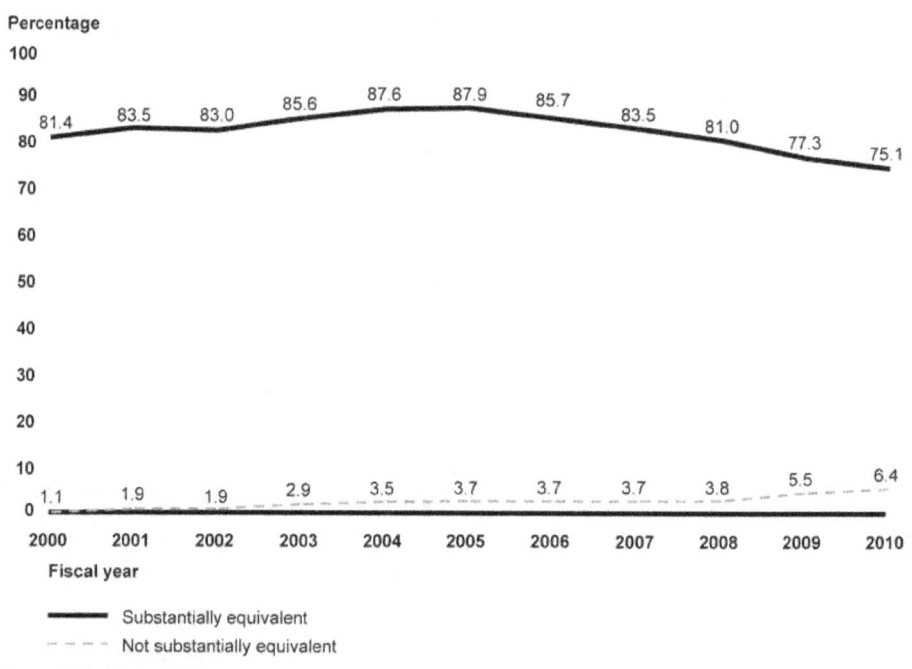

Figure 6: Percentage of FDA Final Decisions That Devices Were Substantially Equivalent or Not Substantially Equivalent for 510(k) Submissions for the Fiscal Year 2000-2010 Cohorts

Source: GAO analysis of FDA data.

Notes: Only 510(k)s that had received a final decision from FDA were included in this analysis.

The percentages for each year do not add to 100 percent because there are other poss ble actions classified as final decisions (e.g., a sponsor's withdrawal of a submission).

FDA Was Inconsistent in Meeting Performance Goals for PMAs While FDA Review Time and Time to Final Decision Generally Increased

For FYs 2003 through 2010, FDA met most of the goals for original PMAs but fell short on most of the goals for expedited PMAs. In addition, FDA review time and time to final decision for both types of PMAs generally increased during this period. Finally, the average number of review cycles increased for certain PMAs while the percentage of PMAs approved after one review cycle generally decreased.

FDA Met Most Goals for Original PMAs but Fell Short of Most Goals for Expedited PMAs from 2003-2010

Since FY 2003, FDA met the original PMA performance goals for four of the seven completed cohorts that had goals in place, but met the goals for only two of the seven expedited PMA cohorts with goals.[35] Specifically, FDA met its Tier 1 performance goals for original PMAs for all three of the completed original PMA cohorts that had such goals in place, with the percentage increasing from 56.8 percent of the FY 2007 cohort to 80.0 percent of the FY 2009 cohort completed on time.[36] (See fig. 7.) While the FY 2010 and 2011 cohorts are still incomplete, FDA is exceeding the goals for those submissions on which it has taken action.[37] FDA's performance had declined steadily in the years immediately before implementation of these goals—from 67.1 percent of the FY 2000 cohort to 34.5 percent of the FY 2006 cohort completed within 180 days.

[35]We treated PMA submissions as meeting the time frame for a given performance goal if they were reviewed within the goal time plus any extension to the goal time that may have been made. The only reason the goal time can be extended is if the sponsor submits a major amendment to the submission on its own initiative (i.e., not solicited by FDA). According to FDA, typical situations that might prompt a sponsor to submit an unsolicited major amendment include when the applicant obtains additional test data related to the safety or effectiveness of the device or obtains new clinical data from a previously unreported study.

[36]PMA performance goals were not designated as Tier 1 or Tier 2 until FY 2008. We have aligned the performance goals in place prior to FY 2008 with the Tier 1 or Tier 2 goals for FYs 2008-2011 based on sharing the same or similar goal time frames. This placement illustrates the increase in the goal percentage over time.

[37]For this analysis, the FY 2010 and 2011 original PMA cohorts were still incomplete. Specifically, for 18.5 percent of the FY 2010 original PMA cohort and 48.8 percent of the FY 2011 cohort, a decision that would permanently stop the review clock for purposes of determining whether FDA met its performance goals had not been made at the time we received FDA's data. As a result, it was too soon to tell what the final results for this cohort would be. It is possible that some of the reviews taking the most time were among those not completed when we received FDA's data. The percentage of original PMAs reviewed within 180 days for these two cohorts may increase or decrease as those reviews are completed.

Figure 7: Percentage of Original PMAs FDA Reviewed within 180 Days for the Fiscal Year 2000-2010 Cohorts

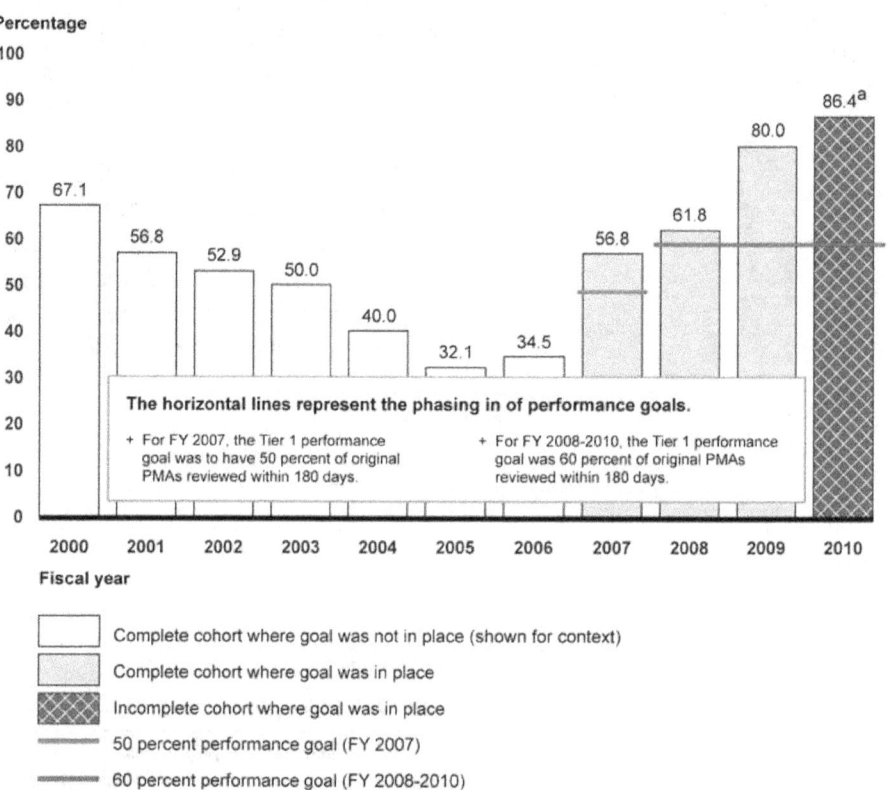

Source: GAO analysis of FDA data.

Notes: Tier 1 and Tier 2 designations refer to the length of time allotted (for the FYs 2008 through 2011 cohorts: 180 days and 295 days, respectively) for FDA to complete its review of original PMA submissions. FDA did not designate PMA performance goals as either Tier 1 or Tier 2 prior to FY 2008. Prior to FY 2006 there were no goals for original PMA submissions. For FY 2006 there was only one goal: 320 days. For FY 2007, the goals for original PMA submissions were 180 days and 320 days. We have aligned the performance goals in place prior to FY 2008 with the Tier 1 and Tier 2 goals for FYs 2008-2011 based on sharing similar time frames. This placement illustrates the increase in the goal percentage over time. If FDA completed its review of a submission in 180 days or less, it met the time frames for both the Tier 1 and Tier 2 goals. If the review was completed in more than 180 days but not more than 320 or 295 days (depending on the cohort), only the time frame for the Tier 2 goal was met. If the review took longer than 320 or 295 days, FDA did not meet the time frame for either goal.

We treated PMA submissions as meeting the time frame for a given performance goal if they were reviewed within the goal time plus any extension to the goal time that may have been made. The only reason the goal time can be extended is if the sponsor submits a major amendment to the submission on its own initiative (i.e., unsolicited by FDA).

aThis analysis includes only those original PMAs for which FDA or the sponsor had made a decision that would permanently stop the review clock for purposes of determining whether FDA met its performance goals (i.e., an approval, approvable, not approvable, withdrawal, or denial); this includes reviews by CBER through September 30, 2011, and reviews by CDRH through December 1, 2011. Submissions without such a decision are not included in the results for each cohort shown above. We considered a cohort to be incomplete if more than 10 percent of submissions had not yet received such a decision. For this analysis, the FY 2010 cohort was still incomplete. Specifically, for 18.5 percent of the FY 2010 original PMA cohort, a decision that would permanently stop the review clock had not been made at the time we received FDA's data. As a result, it was too soon to tell what the final results for this cohort would be. It is possible that some of the reviews taking the most time were among those not completed when we received FDA's data. The percentage of original PMAs reviewed within 180 days for this cohort may increase or decrease as those reviews are completed.

FDA's performance in meeting the Tier 2 performance goals for original PMAs fell short of the goal for three of the four completed cohorts during the years that these goals were in place. FDA met the MDUFMA Tier 2 performance goal (320 days) for the FY 2006 original PMA cohort but not for the FY 2007 cohort, and did not meet the MDUFA Tier 2 performance goal (295 days) for either of the completed cohorts (FYs 2008 and 2009) to which the goal applied (see fig. 8). While the FYs 2010 and 2011 original PMA cohorts are still incomplete, FDA is exceeding the MDUFA Tier 2 goals for those submissions on which it has taken action.[38] FDA's performance varied for original PMA cohorts prior to the years that the Tier 2 goals were in place but was always below the current goal to have 90 percent reviewed within 295 days.

---

[38]For this analysis, the FYs 2010 and 2011 original PMA cohorts were still incomplete. Specifically, for 18.5 percent of the FY 2010 original PMA cohort and 48.8 percent of the FY 2011 cohort, a decision that would permanently stop the review clock for purposes of determining whether FDA met its performance goals had not been made at the time we received FDA's data. As a result, it was too soon to tell what the final results for this cohort would be. It is possible that some of the reviews taking the most time were among those not completed when we received FDA's data. The percentage of original PMAs reviewed within 320 and 295 days for these two cohorts may increase or decrease as those reviews are completed.

Figure 8: Percentage of Original PMAs FDA Reviewed within 320 Days and 295 Days for the Fiscal Year 2000-2010 Cohorts

Original PMAs reviewed within 320 days (MDUFMA Tier 2 goal)

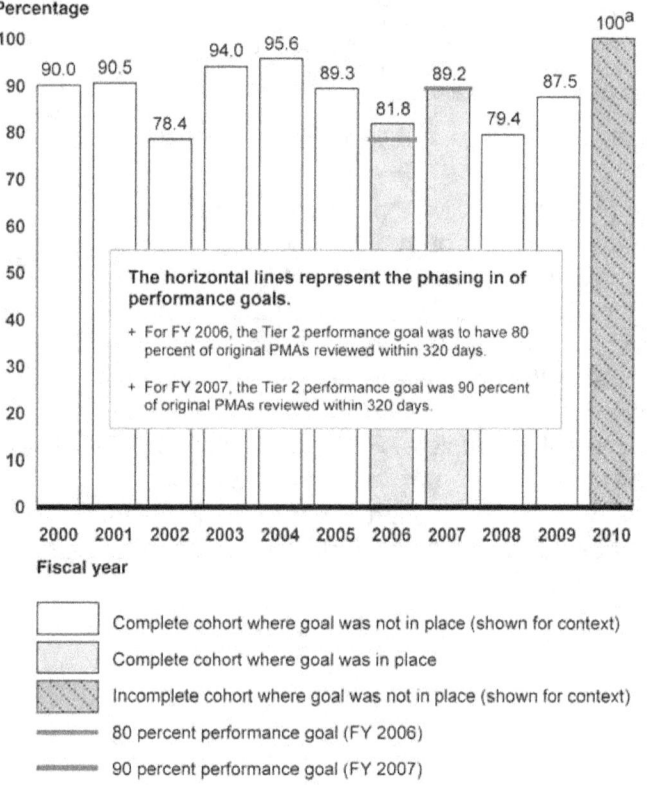

Original PMAs reviewed within 295 days (MDUFA Tier 2 goal)

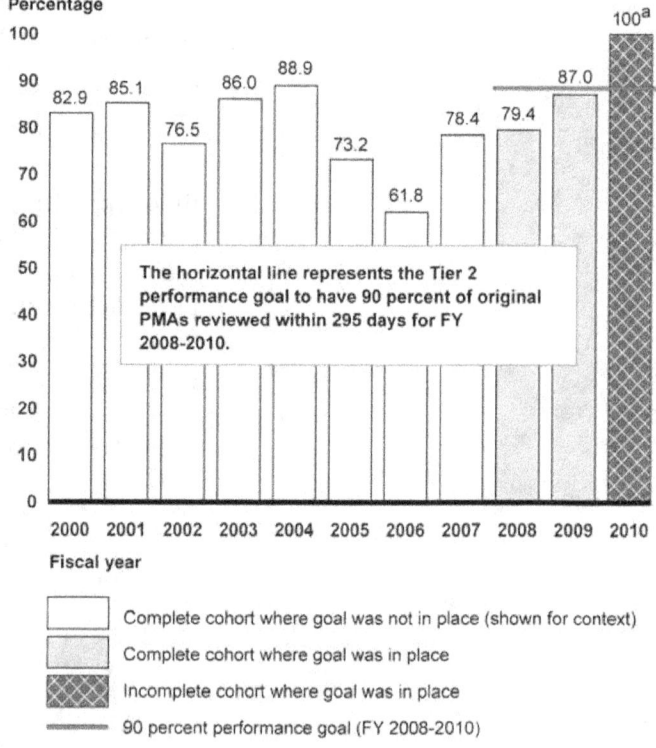

Notes: Tier 1 and Tier 2 designations refer to the length of time allotted (for the FYs 2008-2011 cohorts: 180 days and 295 days, respectively) for FDA to complete its review of original PMA submissions. FDA did not designate PMA performance goals as either Tier 1 or Tier 2 prior to FY 2008. Prior to FY 2006 there were no goals for original PMA submissions. For FY 2006 there was only one goal: 320 days. For FY 2007, the goals for original PMA submissions were 180 days and 320 days. We have aligned the performance goals in place prior to FY 2008 with the Tier 1 and Tier 2 goals for FYs 2008 through 2011 based on sharing similar time frames. This placement illustrates the increase in the goal percentage over time. If FDA completed its review of a submission in 180 days or less, it met the time frames for both the Tier 1 and Tier 2 goals. If the review was completed in more than 180 days but not more than 320 or 295 days (depending on the cohort), only the time frame for the Tier 2 goal was met. If the review took longer than 320 or 295 days, FDA did not meet the time frame for either goal.

We treated PMA submissions as meeting the time frame for a given performance goal if they were reviewed within the goal time plus any extension to the goal time that may have been made. The only reason the goal time can be extended is if the sponsor submits a major amendment to the submission on its own initiative (i.e., unsolicited by FDA).

For expedited PMAs, FDA met the Tier 1 and Tier 2 performance goals for only two of the seven completed cohorts for which the goals were in effect. FDA met the Tier 1 (180-day) goal for only one of the two completed cohorts during the years the goal has been in place, meeting the goal for the FY 2009 cohort but missing it for the FY 2008 cohort (see fig. 9). FDA's performance varied for cohorts prior to the years that the Tier 1 expedited PMA goals were in place but was below the current goal of 50 percent in all but 1 year.

Figure 9: Percentage of Expedited PMAs FDA Reviewed within 180 Days for the Fiscal Year 2000-2010 Cohorts

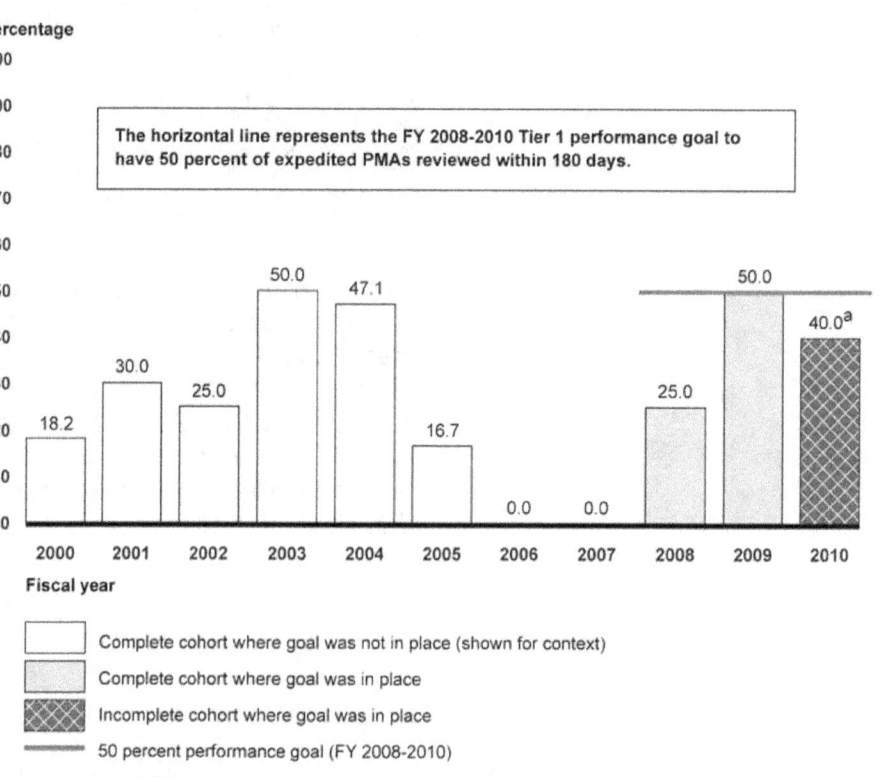

The horizontal line represents the FY 2008-2010 Tier 1 performance goal to have 50 percent of expedited PMAs reviewed within 180 days.

Complete cohort where goal was not in place (shown for context)

Complete cohort where goal was in place

Incomplete cohort where goal was in place

50 percent performance goal (FY 2008-2010)

Source: GAO analysis of FDA data.

Notes: Tier 1 and Tier 2 designations refer to the length of time allotted (for the FYs 2008 through 2011 cohorts: 180 days and 280 days, respectively) for FDA to complete its review of expedited PMA submissions. FDA did not designate PMA performance goals as either Tier 1 or Tier 2 prior to FY 2008. For FYs 2005 through 2007, there was only one goal for expedited PMAs: 300 days. Prior to FY 2005 there were no goals for expedited PMA submissions. We have aligned the performance goal in place prior to FY 2008 with the Tier 2 goal for FYs 2008 through 2011 based on sharing a similar time frame. This placement illustrates the increase in the goal percentage over time. If FDA completed its review of a submission in 180 days or less, it met the time frames for both the Tier 1 and Tier 2 goals. If the review was completed in more than 180 days but not more than 300 or 280 days (depending on the cohort), only the time frame for the Tier 2 goal was met. If the review took longer than 300 or 280 days, FDA did not meet the time frame for either goal.

We treated PMA submissions as meeting the time frame for a given performance goal if they were reviewed within the goal time plus any extension to the goal time that may have been made. The only reason the goal time can be extended is if the sponsor submits a major amendment to the submission on its own initiative (i.e., unsolicited by FDA).

[a]This analysis includes only those expedited PMAs for which FDA or the sponsor had made a decision that would permanently stop the review clock for purposes of determining whether FDA met its performance goals (i.e., an approval, approvable, not approvable, withdrawal, or denial); this includes reviews by CBER through September 30, 2011, and reviews by CDRH through December 1, 2011. Submissions without such a decision are not included in the results for each cohort shown above. We considered a cohort to be incomplete if more than 10 percent of submissions had not yet received such a decision. For this analysis, the FY 2010 expedited PMA cohort was still incomplete. Specifically, for 16.7 percent of the FY 2010 expedited PMA cohort, a decision that would permanently stop the review clock had not been made at the time we received FDA's data. As a result, it was too soon to tell what the final results for this cohort would be. It is possible that some of the reviews taking the most time were among those not completed when we received FDA's data. The percentage of expedited PMAs reviewed within 180 days for this cohort may increase or decrease as those reviews are completed.

FDA's performance in meeting the Tier 2 performance goals for expedited PMAs fell short of the goal for four of the five completed cohorts during the years that these goals were in place. FDA met the MDUFMA Tier 2 performance goal (300 days) for the FY 2005 cohort but not for the FY 2006 or 2007 cohorts, and did not meet the MDUFA Tier 2 performance goal (280 days) for either of the completed cohorts (FY 2008 and 2009) to which the goal applied (see fig. 10). FDA's performance varied for expedited PMA cohorts prior to the years that the Tier 2 goals were in place but always fell below the current goal to have 90 percent reviewed within 280 days.

Figure 10: Percentage of Expedited PMAs FDA Reviewed within 300 Days and 280 Days for the Fiscal Year 2000-2010 Cohorts

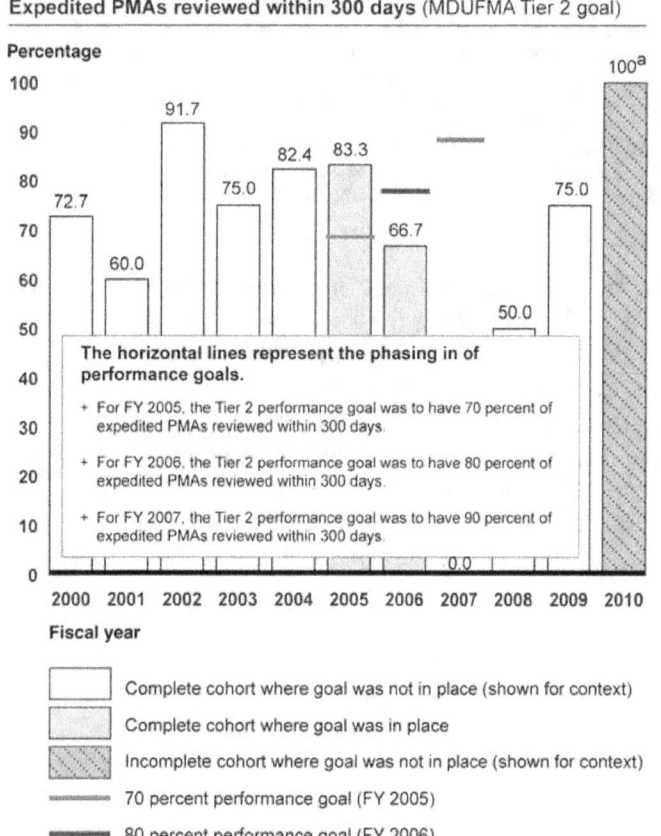

Expedited PMAs reviewed within 300 days (MDUFMA Tier 2 goal)

The horizontal lines represent the phasing in of performance goals.

+ For FY 2005, the Tier 2 performance goal was to have 70 percent of expedited PMAs reviewed within 300 days.

+ For FY 2006, the Tier 2 performance goal was to have 80 percent of expedited PMAs reviewed within 300 days.

+ For FY 2007, the Tier 2 performance goal was to have 90 percent of expedited PMAs reviewed within 300 days.

☐ Complete cohort where goal was not in place (shown for context)
▨ Complete cohort where goal was in place
▨ Incomplete cohort where goal was not in place (shown for context)
— 70 percent performance goal (FY 2005)
— 80 percent performance goal (FY 2006)
— 90 percent performance goal (FY 2007)

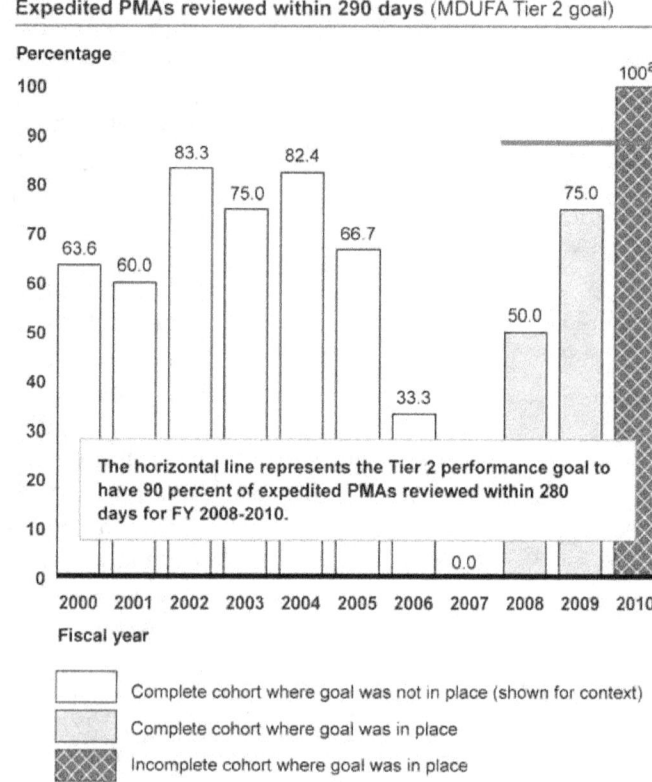

Expedited PMAs reviewed within 290 days (MDUFA Tier 2 goal)

The horizontal line represents the Tier 2 performance goal to have 90 percent of expedited PMAs reviewed within 280 days for FY 2008-2010.

☐ Complete cohort where goal was not in place (shown for context)
▨ Complete cohort where goal was in place
▨ Incomplete cohort where goal was in place
— 90 percent performance goal (FY 2008-2010)

Source: GAO analysis of FDA data.

Notes: Tier 1 and Tier 2 designations refer to the length of time allotted (for the FYs 2008 through 2011 cohorts: 180 days and 280 days, respectively) for FDA to complete its review of expedited PMA submissions. FDA did not designate PMA performance goals as either Tier 1 or Tier 2 prior to FY 2008. For FYs 2005 through 2007, there was only one goal for expedited PMAs: 300 days. Prior to FY 2005 there were no goals for expedited PMA submissions. We have aligned the performance goal in place prior to FY 2008 with the Tier 2 goal for FYs 2008 through 2011 based on sharing a similar time frame. This placement illustrates the increase in the goal percentage over time. If FDA completed its review of a submission in 180 days or less, it met the time frames for both the Tier 1 and Tier 2 goals. If the review was completed in more than 180 days but not more than 300 or 280 days (depending on the cohort), only the time frame for the Tier 2 goal was met. If the review took longer than 300 or 280 days, FDA did not meet the time frame for either goal.

We treated PMA submissions as meeting the time frame for a given performance goal if they were reviewed within the goal time plus any extension to the goal time that may have been made. The only reason the goal time can be extended is if the sponsor submits a major amendment to the submission on its own initiative (i.e., unsolicited by FDA).

FDA Review Time and Time to Final Decision Generally Increased for PMAs from 2003 to 2010

FDA review time for both original and expedited PMAs was highly variable but generally increased across our analysis period, while time to final decision also increased for original PMAs. Specifically, average FDA review time for original PMAs increased from 211 days in the FY 2003 cohort (the first year that user fees were in effect) to 264 days in the FY 2008 cohort, then fell in the FY 2009 cohort to 217 days (see fig. 11). When we added off-the-clock time (during which FDA waited for the sponsor to provide additional information or correct deficiencies in the submission), average time to final decision for the FYs 2003 through 2008 cohorts fluctuated from year to year but trended upward from 462 days for the FY 2003 cohort to 627 days for the FY 2008 cohort.[39]

---

[39]The FY 2009 original PMA cohort is complete for purposes of calculating FDA review time but incomplete for the calculation of time to final decision because some submissions in the cohort have received a decision ending a review cycle (e.g., approvable letter) and permanently stopping the review clock for purposes of determining whether FDA met its performance goals, but have not yet received a final decision such as approval or denial that would end the review process.

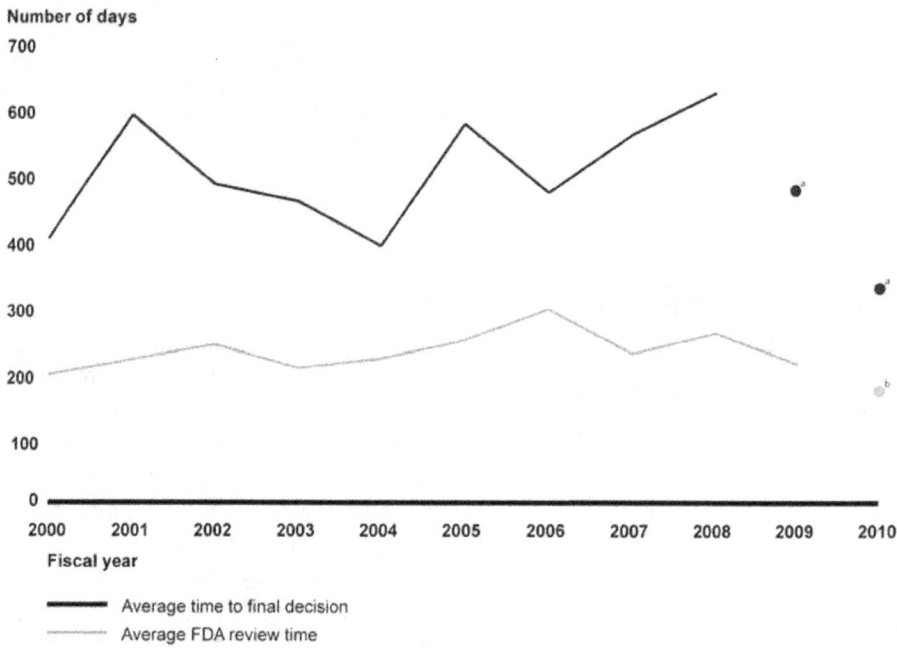

Figure 11: Average FDA Review Time and Average Time to Final Decision for Original PMAs in the Fiscal Year 2000-2010 Cohorts

Source: GAO analysis of FDA data.

Note: FDA review time refers to the time that FDA spends reviewing a submission and therefore excludes any time the sponsor may spend responding to FDA requests for additional information. Time to final decision includes both the time FDA spends reviewing a submission and the time the sponsor may spend responding to any FDA action.

[a]The analysis of time to final decision includes only those original PMAs for which FDA or the sponsor had made a final decision (i.e., a decision that ends the review process such as an approval, denial, or withdrawal); this includes reviews by CBER through September 30, 2011, and reviews by CDRH through December 1, 2011. Submissions without a final decision are not included in the results for each cohort shown above. We considered a cohort to be incomplete if more than 10 percent of submissions had not yet received a final decision. For this analysis, the FYs 2009-2010 original PMA cohorts were still incomplete. Specifically, 22 percent of the FY 2009 original PMA cohort and 46.3 percent of the FY 2010 cohort had not yet received a final decision. As a result, it was too soon to tell what the final results for this cohort would be. It is possible that some of the reviews taking the most time were among those not completed when we received FDA's data. The average time to final decision for these two cohorts may increase or decrease as those reviews are completed.

bThe analysis of FDA review time includes only those original PMAs for which FDA or the sponsor had made a decision that would permanently stop the review clock for purposes of determining whether FDA met its performance goals (i.e., an approval, approvable, not approvable, withdrawal, or denial); this includes reviews by CBER through September 30, 2011, and reviews by CDRH through December 1, 2011. Submissions without such a decision are not included in the results for each cohort shown above. We considered a cohort to be incomplete if more than 10 percent of submissions had not yet received such a decision. For this analysis, the FY 2010 original PMA cohort was still incomplete. Specifically, for 18.5 percent of the FY 2010 original PMA cohort, a decision that would permanently stop the review clock had not been made at the time we received FDA's data. As a result, it was too soon to tell what the final results for this cohort would be. It is possible that some of the reviews taking the most time were among those not completed when we received FDA's data. The average FDA review time for this cohort may increase or decrease as those reviews are completed.

The results for expedited PMAs fluctuated even more dramatically than for original PMAs—likely due to the small number of submissions (about 7 per year on average). Average FDA review time for expedited PMAs generally increased over the period that user fees have been in effect, from 241 days for the FY 2003 cohort to 356 days for the FY 2008 cohort, then fell to 245 days for the FY 2009 cohort (see fig. 12). The average time to final decision for expedited PMAs was highly variable but overall declined somewhat during this period, from 704 days for the FY 2003 cohort to 545 days for the FY 2009 cohort.

Figure 12: Average FDA Review Time and Average Time to Final Decision for Expedited PMAs in the Fiscal Year 2000-2010 Cohorts

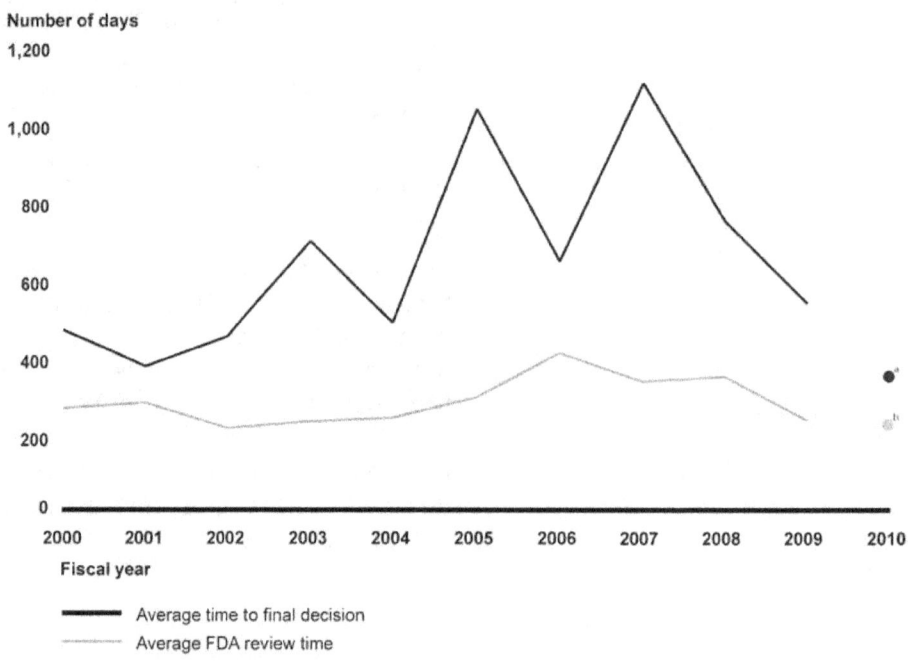

Number of days

Fiscal year

—— Average time to final decision

------- Average FDA review time

Source: GAO analysis of FDA data.

Note: FDA review time refers to the time that FDA spends reviewing a submission and therefore excludes any time the sponsor may spend responding to FDA requests for additional information. Time to final decision includes both the time FDA spends reviewing a submission and the time the sponsor may spend responding to any FDA action.

[a]The analysis of time to final decision includes only those expedited PMAs for which FDA or the sponsor had made a final decision (i.e., a decision that ends the review process such as an approval, denial, or withdrawal); this includes reviews by CBER through September 30, 2011, and reviews by CDRH through December 1, 2011. Submissions without a final decision are not included in the results for each cohort shown above. We considered a cohort to be incomplete if more than 10 percent of submissions had not yet received a final decision. For this analysis, the FY 2010 expedited PMA cohort was still incomplete. Specifically, 33 percent of the FY 2010 expedited PMA cohort had not yet received a final decision. As a result, it was too soon to tell what the final results for this cohort would be. It is possible that some of the reviews taking the most time were among those not completed when we received FDA's data. The average time to final decision for this cohort may increase or decrease as those reviews are completed.

The Average Number of Review Cycles Increased for Certain PMAs While the Percentage of PMAs Approved after One Review Cycle Generally Decreased

The average number of review cycles per original PMA increased 27.5 percent from 1.82 in the FY 2003 cohort (the first year that user fees were in effect) to 2.32 cycles in the FY 2008 cohort. For expedited PMAs, the average number of review cycles per submission was fairly steady at approximately 2.5 cycles until the FY 2004 cohort, then peaked at 4.0 in the FY 2006 cohort before decreasing back to 2.5 cycles in the FY 2009 cohort. We found nearly identical trends when we examined the subsets of original and expedited PMAs that received a final FDA decision of approval.

In addition, the percentage of original PMAs receiving a decision of approval at the end of the first review cycle fluctuated from FYs 2003 through 2009 but generally decreased—from 16 percent in the FY 2003 cohort to 9.8 percent in the FY 2009 cohort. Similarly, the percentage receiving a first-cycle approvable decision decreased from 12 percent in the FY 2003 cohort to 2.4 percent in the FY 2009 cohort. The percentage of expedited PMAs receiving first-cycle approval fluctuated from year to year, from 0 percent in 5 of the years we examined to a maximum of 25 percent in FY 2008.

The percentage of original PMAs that ultimately received approval from FDA fluctuated from year to year but exhibited an overall decrease for the completed cohorts from FYs 2003 through 2008. Specifically, 74.0 percent of original PMAs in the FY 2003 cohort were ultimately approved, compared to 68.8 percent of the FY 2008 cohort. The percentage of expedited PMAs that were ultimately approved varied significantly from FYs 2003 through 2009, from a low of 0 percent in the FY 2007 cohort to a high of 100 percent in the FY 2006 cohort.

Stakeholders Noted Issues with the Medical Device Review Process; FDA Is Taking Steps That May Address Many of These Issues

The industry groups and consumer advocacy groups we interviewed noted a number of issues related to FDA's review of medical device submissions. The most commonly mentioned issue raised by industry and consumer advocacy stakeholder groups was insufficient communication between FDA and stakeholders throughout the review process. Industry stakeholders also noted a lack of predictability and consistency in reviews and an increase in time to final decision. Consumer advocacy group stakeholders noted issues related to inadequate assurance of the safety and effectiveness of approved or cleared devices. FDA is taking steps that may address many of these issues.

Stakeholders Cite Insufficient Communication between FDA and Stakeholders throughout the Review Process

Most of the three industry and four consumer advocacy group stakeholders that we interviewed told us that there is insufficient communication between FDA and stakeholders throughout the review process. For example, four stakeholders noted that FDA does not clearly communicate to stakeholders the regulatory standards that it uses to evaluate submissions. In particular, industry stakeholders noted problems with the regulatory guidance documents issued by FDA. These stakeholders noted that these guidance documents are often unclear, out of date, and not comprehensive. Stakeholders also noted that after sponsors submit their applications to FDA, insufficient communication from FDA prevents sponsors from learning about deficiencies in their submissions early in FDA's review. According to one of these stakeholders, if FDA communicated these deficiencies earlier in the process, sponsors would be able to correct them and would be less likely to receive a request for additional information. Two consumer advocacy group stakeholders also noted that FDA does not sufficiently seek patient input during reviews. One stakeholder noted that it is important for FDA to incorporate patient perspectives into its reviews of medical devices because patients might weigh the benefits and risks of a certain device differently than FDA reviewers.

FDA has taken or plans to take several steps that may address issues with the frequency and quality of its communications with stakeholders, including issuing new guidance documents, improving the guidance development process, and enhancing interactions between FDA and stakeholders during reviews. For example, in December 2011, FDA released draft guidance about the regulatory framework, policies, and practices underlying FDA's 510(k) review in order to enhance the transparency of this program.[40] In addition, FDA implemented a tracking system and released a standard operating procedure (SOP) for developing guidance documents for medical device reviews to provide greater clarity, predictability, and efficiency in this process.[41] FDA also created a new staff position to oversee the guidance development process. Additionally, according to an overview of recent FDA actions to improve its device review programs, FDA is currently enhancing its interactive review process for medical device reviews by establishing performance goals for early and substantive interactions between FDA and sponsors during reviews.[42] This overview also notes that FDA is currently working with a coalition of patient advocacy groups on establishing mechanisms for obtaining reliable information on patient perspectives during medical device reviews.[43]

Industry Stakeholders Report a Lack of Predictability and Consistency in Reviews

The three industry stakeholders that we interviewed also told us that there is a lack of predictability and consistency in FDA's reviews of device submissions. For example, two stakeholders noted that review criteria sometimes change after a sponsor submits an application. In particular, one of these stakeholders noted that criteria sometimes change when the FDA reviewer assigned to the submission changes during the review. Additionally, stakeholders noted that there is sometimes inconsistent

---

[40]See U.S. Department of Health and Human Services, Food and Drug Administration, *Draft Guidance for Industry and Food and Drug Administration Staff. The 510(k) Program: Evaluating Substantial Equivalence in Premarket Notifications [510(k)]* (Silver Spring, Md.: Dec. 27, 2011).

[41]See U.S. Department of Health and Human Services, Food and Drug Administration, *CDRH Guidance Development* (Silver Spring, Md.: Aug. 1, 2011).

[42]See U.S. Department of Health and Human Services, Food and Drug Administration, *Medical Device Premarket Programs: An Overview of FDA Actions* (Silver Spring, Md.: Oct. 19, 2011). Interactive review—which was established following the 2007 reauthorization of the medical device user fee program—was created to formalize a process to encourage and facilitate communication between FDA and sponsors during reviews.

[43]Additionally, FDA recently issued draft guidance regarding the factors that FDA considers when making benefit-risk determinations in order to increase the transparency of these determinations. See U.S. Department of Health and Human Services, Food and Drug Administration, *Draft Guidance for Industry and Food and Drug Administration Staff. Factors to Consider when Making Benefit-Risk Determinations in Medical Device Premarket Review* (Silver Spring, Md.: Aug. 15, 2011). According to FDA, the criteria in this guidance take a patient-centric approach by calling for the consideration of patients' tolerance for risk.

application of criteria across review divisions or across individual reviewers. Stakeholders noted that enhanced training for reviewers and enhanced supervisory oversight could help resolve inconsistencies in reviews and increase predictability for sponsors.

In the two internal assessments of its device review programs that FDA released in August 2010, the agency found that insufficient predictability in its review programs was a significant problem.[44] FDA has taken steps that may address issues with the predictability and consistency of its reviews of device submissions, including issuing new SOPs for reviews and enhancing training for FDA staff. For example, in June 2011, FDA issued an SOP to standardize the practice of quickly issuing written notices to sponsors to inform them about changes in FDA's regulatory expectations for medical device submissions.[45] FDA also recently developed an SOP to assure greater consistency in the review of device submissions when review staff change during the review.[46] Additionally, in April 2010, FDA began a reviewer certification program for new FDA

---

[44]See U.S. Department of Health and Human Services, Food and Drug Administration, *510(k) Working Group: Preliminary Report and Recommendations* (Silver Spring, Md.: August 2010) and U.S. Department of Health and Human Services, Food and Drug Administration, *Task Force on the Utilization of Science in Regulatory Decision Making, Preliminary Report and Recommendations* (Silver Spring, Md.: August 2010). FDA identified several causes of the issues noted in these assessments, including very high reviewer and manager turnover at CDRH; insufficient training for staff and industry; extremely high ratios of front-line supervisors to employees; insufficient oversight by managers; CDRH's rapidly growing workload, caused by the increasing complexity of devices and the number of submissions reviewed; unnecessary and/or inconsistent data requirements imposed on device sponsors; insufficient guidance for industry; and poor-quality submissions from industry.

[45]See U.S. Department of Health and Human Services, Food and Drug Administration, *CDRH Standard Operating Procedure for "Notice to Industry" Letters* (Silver Spring, Md.: June 14, 2011). The SOP provides a streamlined, systematic process for communicating with industry via the guidance process and other means, as appropriate. Notice to Industry letters are short communications that describe, at a very high level, changes to scientific data requirements and FDA's reasons for those changes. Some of these letters may constitute guidance, while others will not. Because these letters are short and are overseen by upper management at the Center, they can be developed and released in roughly 3 weeks. FDA posts these letters on its website and also uses additional methods for distributing the letters to stakeholders.

[46]See U.S. Department of Health and Human Services, Food and Drug Administration, *SOP: Management of Review Staff Changes During the Review of a Premarket Submission* (Silver Spring, Md.: Dec. 27, 2011).

reviewers designed to improve the consistency of reviews.[47] According to the overview of recent FDA actions to improve its device review programs, FDA also plans to implement an experiential learning program for new reviewers to give them a better understanding of how medical devices are designed, manufactured, and used.[48]

Industry Stakeholders Note an Increase in Time to Final Decision

The three industry stakeholders we interviewed told us that the time to final decision for device submissions has increased in recent years. This is consistent with our analysis, which showed that the average time to final decision has increased for completed 510(k) and original PMA cohorts since FY 2003. Additionally, stakeholders noted that FDA has increased the number of requests for additional information, which our analysis also shows. Stakeholders told us they believe the additional information being requested is not always critical for the review of the submission. Additional information requests increase the time to final decision but not necessarily the FDA review time because FDA stops the review clock when it requests additional information from sponsors. Two of the stakeholders stated that reviewers may be requesting additional information more often due to a culture of increased risk aversion at FDA or because they want to stop the review clock in order to meet performance goals.

According to FDA, the most significant contributor to the increased number of requests for additional information—and therefore increased time to final decision—is the poor quality of submissions received from sponsors. In July 2011, FDA released an analysis it conducted of review times under the 510(k) program.[49] According to FDA, in over 80 percent of the reviews studied for this analysis, reviewers asked for additional

---

[47]See U.S. Department of Health and Human Services, Food and Drug Administration, *Driving Biomedical Innovation: Initiatives to Improve Products for Patients* (Silver Spring, Md.: October 2011). The reviewer certification program includes up to 18 months of training on specific core competencies through online training modules, instructor-led courses, and practical experience.

[48]The experiential learning program will include visits to academic institutions, manufacturers, research organizations, and health care facilities to provide new reviewers with a broader view of the regulatory process for medical devices.

[49]See U.S. Department of Health and Human Services, Food and Drug Administration, *Analysis of Premarket Review Times Under the 510(k) Program* (Silver Spring, Md.: July 2011).

information from sponsors due to problems with the quality of the submission.[50] FDA officials told us that sending a request for additional information is often the only option for reviewers besides issuing a negative decision to the sponsor. FDA's analysis also found that 8 percent of its requests for additional information during the first review cycle were inappropriate. Requests for additional information were deemed inappropriate if FDA requested additional information or data for a 510(k) that (1) were not justified, (2) were not permissible as a matter of federal law or FDA policy, or (3) were unnecessary to make a substantial equivalence determination. FDA has taken steps that may address issues with the number of inappropriate requests for additional information. For example, the overview of recent FDA actions indicates the agency is developing an SOP for requests for additional information that clarifies when these requests can be made for 510(k)s, the types of requests that can be made, and the management level at which the decision must be made.

Consumer Advocacy Group Stakeholders Suggest That FDA Provides Inadequate Assurance of the Safety and Effectiveness of Approved or Cleared Devices

Three of the four consumer advocacy group stakeholders with whom we spoke stated that FDA is not adequately ensuring the safety and effectiveness of the devices it approves or clears for marketing. One of these stakeholders told us that FDA prioritizes review speed over safety and effectiveness. Two stakeholders also noted that the standards FDA uses to approve or clear devices are lower than the standards that FDA uses to approve drugs, particularly for the 510(k) program. Two stakeholders also expressed concern that devices reviewed under the 510(k) program are not always sufficiently similar to their predicates and that devices whose predicates are recalled due to safety concerns do not have to be reassessed to ensure that they are safe. Finally, three stakeholders told us that FDA does not gather enough data on long-term device safety and effectiveness through methods such as postmarket analysis and device tracking.

These issues are similar to those raised elsewhere, such as a public meeting to discuss the reauthorization of the medical device user fee program, a congressional hearing, and an Institute of Medicine (IOM)

---

[50]Quality problems included (1) inadequate device description, (2) discrepancies throughout the submission, (3) problems with the indications for use, (4) failure to follow or otherwise address current guidance documents or recognized standards, (5) lack of performance data, and (6) lack of clinical data.

report. For example, during a September 14, 2010, public meeting to discuss the reauthorization, consumer advocacy groups—including two of those we interviewed for our report—urged the inclusion of safety and effectiveness improvements in the reauthorization, including raising premarket review standards for devices and increasing postmarket surveillance.[51] Additionally, during an April 13, 2011, congressional hearing, another consumer advocacy group expressed concerns about FDA's 510(k) review process and recalls of high-risk devices that were cleared through this process.[52] Finally, in July 2011, IOM released a report summarizing the results of an independent evaluation of the 510(k) program. FDA had requested that IOM conduct this evaluation to determine whether the 510(k) program optimally protects patients and promotes innovation. IOM concluded that clearance of a 510(k) based on substantial equivalence to a predicate device is not a determination that the cleared device is safe or effective.[53]

FDA has taken or plans to take steps that may address issues with the safety and effectiveness of approved and cleared devices, including evaluating the 510(k) program and developing new data systems. For example, FDA analyzed the safety of 510(k) devices cleared on the basis of multiple predicates by investigating an apparent association between

---

[51]See U.S. Department of Health and Human Services, Food and Drug Administration, *Medical Device User Fee Program Public Meeting* (Hyattsville, Md.: Sept. 14, 2010).

[52]See *A Delicate Balance: FDA and the Reform of the Medical Device Approval Process, Hearing Before the Special Committee on Aging, United States Senate,* 112th Cong. (2011) (statement of Diana Zuckerman, President, National Research Center for Women and Families, Cancer Prevention and Treatment Fund).

[53]See Institute of Medicine of the National Academies, *Medical Devices and the Public's Health, The FDA 510(k) Clearance Process at 35 Years* (Washington, D.C.: July 29, 2011). IOM concluded that the standard for assessing substantial equivalence to a predicate device for clearance under the 510(k) program generally does not require evidence of safety or effectiveness of a device. Therefore, IOM concluded that FDA cannot evaluate the safety and effectiveness of devices as long as the standard for clearance is substantial equivalence, as directed in statute. IOM also concluded that available information on postmarket performance of devices does not provide sufficient information about potential harm or lack of effectiveness to be a useful source of data on the safety and effectiveness of marketed devices. IOM does not believe, however, that there is a public-health crisis related to unsafe or ineffective medical devices. See also GAO, *Medical Devices: FDA Should Take Steps to Ensure That High-Risk Device Types Are Approved through the Most Stringent Premarket Review Process,* GAO-09-190 (Washington, D.C.: Jan. 15, 2009).

these devices and increased reports of adverse events.[54] FDA concluded that no clear relationship exists. FDA also conducted a public meeting to discuss the recommendations proposed in the IOM report in September 2011.[55] FDA is also developing a device identification system that will allow FDA to better track devices that are distributed to patients, as well as an electronic reporting system that will assist with tracking and analyzing adverse events in marketed devices.[56]

Concluding Observations

While FDA has met most of the goals for the time frames within which the agency was to review and take action on 510(k) and PMA device submissions, the time that elapses before a final decision has been increasing. This is particularly true for 510(k) submissions, which comprise the bulk of FDA device reviews. Stakeholders we spoke with point to a number of issues that the agency could consider in addressing the cause of these time increases. FDA tracks and reports the time to final decision in its annual reports to Congress on the medical device user fee program, and its own reports reveal the same pattern we found. In its July 2011 analysis of 510(k) submissions, FDA concluded that reviewers asked for additional information from sponsors—thus stopping the clock on FDA's review time while the total time to reach a final decision continued to elapse—mainly due to problems with the quality of the submission. FDA is taking steps that may address the increasing time to final decision. It is important for the agency to monitor the impact of those steps in ensuring that safe and effective medical devices are reaching the market in a timely manner.

[54]See U.S. Department of Health and Human Services, Food and Drug Administration, *Medical Device Reporting (MDR) Rate in 510(k) Cleared Devices Using Multiple Predicates* (Silver Spring, Md.: Oct. 14, 2011). A sponsor may cite more than one predicate device in a submission for several reasons. For example, multiple devices, each with its own predicate, may be bundled together into one submission. A sponsor may also cite multiple predicates when a single device combines the functions of more than one device.

[55]See 76 *Fed. Reg.* 50,230 (Aug. 12, 2011).

[56]FDA held a public workshop on the adoption, implementation, and use of unique device identifiers in various health-related electronic data systems in September 2011. See 76 *Fed. Reg.* 43,691 (July 21, 2011). According to FDA's plan of action, FDA is also currently developing proposed regulations for the unique device identifier system.

Agency Comments

HHS reviewed a draft of this report and provided written comments, which are reprinted in appendix III. HHS generally agreed with our findings and noted that FDA has identified some of the same performance trends in its annual reports to Congress. HHS noted that because the total time to final decision includes the time industry incurs in responding to FDA's concerns, FDA and industry bear shared responsibility for the increase in this time and will need to work together to achieve improvement. HHS also noted that in January 2011, FDA announced 25 specific actions that the agency would take to improve the predictability, consistency, and transparency of its premarket medical device review programs. Since then, HHS stated, FDA has taken or is taking actions designed to create a culture change toward greater transparency, interaction, collaboration, and the appropriate balancing of benefits and risk; ensure predictable and consistent recommendations, decision making, and application of the least burdensome principle; and implement efficient processes and use of resources. HHS also provided technical comments, which we incorporated as appropriate.

As agreed with your office, unless you publicly announce the contents of this report earlier, we plan no further distribution until 30 days from the report date. At that time, we will send copies of this report to the Secretary of Health and Human Services, the Commissioner of FDA, and other interested parties. In addition, the report will be available at no charge on the GAO website at http://www.gao.gov.

If you or your staff have any questions about this report, please contact me at (202) 512-7114 or crossem@gao.gov. Contact points for our Offices of Congressional Relations and Public Affairs may be found on the last page of this report. GAO staff who made key contributions to this report are listed in appendix IV.

Marcia Crosse
Director, Health Care

Table 4: FDA Premarket Notification (510(k)) Review Performance, FYs 2000–2011

Fiscal year cohorts	Prior to implementation of the Medical Device User Fee and Modernization Act of 2002 (MDUFMA)			Period covered by MDUFMA					Period covered by the Medical Device User Fee Amendments of 2007 (MDUFA)			
	2000	2001	2002	2003	2004	2005	2006	2007	2008	2009	2010	2011[a]
Total number of 510(k) submissions	4,242	4,294	4,365	4,292	3,711	3,713	3,914	3,714	3,901	4,153	3,938	3,878
Number of 510(k) submissions with a final FDA decision	4,242	4,294	4,365	4,292	3,711	3,713	3,914	3,713	3,899	4,148	3,853	2,366
Number reviewed in ≤ 90 days[b]	3,391	3,279	3,411	3,299	3,121	3,381	3,569	3,364	3,651	3,737	3,530	2,300
Percentage reviewed in ≤ 90 days[b]	79.9	76.4	78.1	76.9	84.1	91.1	91.2	90.6	93.6	90.1	91.6	97.2
Tier 1 goal percentage[c]	—	—	—	—	—	75	75	80	90	90	90	90
Met Tier 1 goal[d]	n/a	n/a	n/a	n/a	n/a	Yes	Yes	Yes	Yes	Yes	Yes[e]	Yes[e]
Number reviewed in ≤ 150 days[b]	3,796	3,773	3,863	3,773	3,535	3,623	3,799	3,591	3,835	4,049	3,795	2,361
Percentage reviewed in ≤ 150 days[b]	89.5	87.9	88.5	87.9	95.3	97.6	97.1	96.7	98.4	97.6	98.5	99.8
Tier 2 goal percentage[c]	—	—	—	—	—	—	—	—	98	98	98	98
Met Tier 2 goal[d]	n/a	n/a	n/a	n/a	n/a	n/a	n/a	n/a	Yes	Yes	Yes[e]	Yes[e]
Average number of review cycles per submission[f]	1.38	1.43	1.39	1.47	1.53	1.61	1.69	1.78	1.83	1.94	2.04	1.64
Of first-cycle decisions, percentage that were substantially equivalent (SE)	54.1	53.8	55.7	54.0	52.1	47.7	42.2	36.6	33.3	26.2	20.0	21.2
Among 510(k) submissions with a final decision, percentage of final decisions that were:												
Substantially equivalent (SE)	81.4	83.5	83.0	85.6	87.6	87.9	85.7	83.5	81.0	77.3	75.1	87.2
Not substantially equivalent (NSE)	1.1	1.9	1.9	2.9	3.5	3.7	3.7	3.7	3.8	5.5	6.4	2.4
Withdrawn	0.1	0.1	0.2	0.3	0.1	0.2	0.1	0.2	0.1	0.2	0.3	0.1
Other	17.4	14.5	14.9	11.3	8.7	8.2	10.4	12.7	15.1	16.9	18.3	10.4
Average FDA review time (in days) for 510(k) submissions that were not reviewed within 150 days	195	201	201	197	195	186	221	228	259	282	226	176

Fiscal year cohorts	Prior to implementation of the Medical Device User Fee and Modernization Act of 2002 (MDUFMA)			Period covered by MDUFMA					Period covered by the Medical Device User Fee Amendments of 2007 (MDUFA)			
	2000	2001	2002	2003	2004	2005	2006	2007	2008	2009	2010	2011[a]
Average time to final decision (in days) for 510(k) submissions that were not reviewed within 150 days	295	302	300	306	325	374	426	429	457	460	377	269

Source: GAO analysis of Food and Drug Administration (FDA) data.

Note: A review cohort includes all the medical device submissions relating to a particular performance goal that were submitted in a given fiscal year. For example, all 510(k)s received by FDA from October 1, 2010, to September 30, 2011, make up the 510(k) review cohort for FY 2011. Cohorts were considered complete if fewer than 10 percent of submissions were still under review at the time we received FDA's data. All cohorts except FY 2011 were complete for the purposes of our analysis. As a result, it was too soon to tell what the final results for this cohort would be.

[a]Approximately 39 percent of 510(k)s received in fiscal year (FY) 2011 were still under review at the time we received FDA's data, which cover reviews by CDRH through October 26, 2011, and reviews by CBER through December 23, 2011. As a result, it was too soon to tell what the final results for this cohort would be. It is possible that some of the reviews taking the most time were among those not completed when we received FDA's data. The percentage of 510(k)s reviewed within 90 days and within 150 days for the FY 2011 cohort may increase or decrease as those reviews are completed. The number of 510(k)s reviewed within 90 and 150 days and the average number of review cycles for the FY 2011 cohort may increase as those reviews are completed but will not decrease.

[b]Only 510(k)s that had received a final decision from FDA were used to determine the number and percentage of 510(k)s reviewed within 90 days and within 150 days.

[c]Fiscal years for which there was no corresponding 510(k) performance goal are denoted with a dash (—).

[d]"n/a" denotes not applicable. In these years, there was no corresponding 510(k) performance goal and therefore no determination of whether the goal was met.

[e]These results may change as the remaining 510(k) submissions for the FY 2010 and FY 2011 cohorts receive final decisions.

[f]Cycles that were currently in progress at the time we received FDA's data were included in this analysis. The average number of review cycles for the FY 2011 cohort may increase as those reviews are completed but will not decrease.

Table 5: FDA Premarket Approval (PMA) Review Performance for Original PMAs, FYs 2000–2011

Fiscal years	Pre-MDUFMA			MDUFMA					MDUFA			
	2000	2001	2002	2003	2004	2005	2006	2007	2008	2009	2010[a]	2011[a]
Total number of submissions	73	75	51	50	45	57	55	37	34	41	54	43
Number reviewed in ≤ 180 days[b]	47	42	27	25	18	18	19	21	21	32	38	20
Percentage reviewed in ≤ 180 days[b]	67.1	56.8	52.9	50.0	40.0	32.1	34.5	56.8	61.8	80.0	86.4	90.9
Tier 1 goal percentage[c]	—	—	—	—	—	—	—	50	60	60	60	60
Met Tier 1 goal[d]	n/a	n/a	n/a	n/a	n/a	n/a	n/a	n/a	Yes	Yes	Yes[e]	Yes[e]
Number reviewed in ≤ 320 days[b]	63	67	40	47	43	50	45	33	27	35	44	22
Percentage reviewed in ≤ 320 days[b]	90.0	90.5	78.4	94.0	95.6	89.3	81.8	89.2	79.4	87.5	100.0	100.0
Tier 2 goal percentage[c]	—	—	—	—	—	—	80	90	—	—	—	—
Met Tier 2 goal[d]	n/a	n/a	n/a	n/a	n/a	n/a	Yes	No	n/a	n/a	n/a	n/a
Number reviewed in ≤ 295 days[b]	58	63	39	43	40	41	34	29	27	35	44	22
Percentage reviewed in ≤ 295 days[b]	82.9	85.1	76.5	86.0	88.9	73.2	61.8	78.4	79.4	87.5	100.0	100.0
Tier 2 goal percentage[c]	—	—	—	—	—	—	—	—	90	90	90	90
Met Tier 2 goal[d]	n/a	n/a	n/a	n/a	n/a	n/a	n/a	n/a	No	No	Yes[e]	Yes[e]
Average number of review cycles per submission[f]	1.77	2.05	2.16	1.82	1.98	2.54	2.40	2.51	2.32	2.12[g]	2.04	1.58
Of first-cycle decisions, percentage that were approval	15.1	17.3	9.8	16.0	8.9	8.8	21.8	8.1	5.9	9.8	7.4	9.3
Among original PMAs with a final decision, percentage of final decisions that were:												
Approval [g]	61.6	69.3	76.5	74.0	79.5	71.4	90.4	70.6	68.8	56.3	82.8	93.3
Denial[g]	0.0	0.0	0.0	0.0	0.0	0.0	0.0	0.0	0.0	0.0	0.0	0.0
Withdrawal[g]	31.5	28.0	23.5	26.0	20.5	28.6	9.6	29.4	31.3	43.8	17.2	6.7
Average FDA review time (in days) for original PMAs that were not reviewed within 295 days[b]	383	468	451	333	368	342	447	422	584	571	—[h]	—[h]
Average time to final decision (in days) for original PMAs that were not reviewed within 295 days[g]	752	1006	688	591	775	727	679	645	923	823	—[h]	—[h]

Source: GAO analysis of FDA data.

Notes: A review cohort includes all the medical device submissions relating to a particular performance goal that were submitted in a given fiscal year. For example, all original PMAs received by FDA from October 1, 2010, to September 30, 2011, make up the original PMA review cohort for FY 2011. Cohorts were considered complete if fewer than 10 percent of submissions were still under review at the time we received FDA's data.

We treated PMA submissions as meeting the time frame for a given performance goal if they were reviewed within the goal time plus any extension to the goal time that may have been made. The only reason the goal time can be extended is if the sponsor submits a major amendment to the submission on its own initiative (i.e., unsolicited by FDA).

[a]The FYs 2010 and 2011 original PMA cohorts were considered still incomplete. Specifically, for 18.5 percent of the FY 2010 original PMA cohort and 48.8 percent of the FY 2011 cohort, FDA had not yet made a decision that would permanently stop the review clock for purposes of determining whether FDA met its performance goals (i.e., an approval, approvable, not approvable, withdrawal, or denial) at the time we received FDA's data; this includes reviews by CBER through September 30, 2011, and reviews by CDRH through December 1, 2011. As a result, it was too soon to tell what the final results for these cohorts would be. It is poss ble that some of the reviews taking the most time were among those not completed when we received FDA's data. The percentage of original PMAs reviewed within 180 days for the FY 2010 and FY 2011 cohorts may increase or decrease as those reviews are completed; the number reviewed within 180 days and the number and percentage reviewed within 320 days and within 295 days may decrease as those reviews are completed.

[b]Only original PMAs that had received a decision permanently stopping the review clock were used to determine the number and percentage of original PMAs reviewed within 180 days, within 320 days, and within 295 days.

[c]Fiscal years for which there was no corresponding original PMA performance goal are denoted with a dash (—).

[d]"n/a" denotes not applicable. In these years, there was no corresponding original PMA performance goal and therefore no determination of whether the goal was met.

[e]These results may change as the remaining original PMA submissions for the FY 2010 and FY 2011 cohorts receive decisions that permanently stop the review clock for purposes of determining whether FDA met its performance goals.

[f]Cycles that were currently in progress at the time we received FDA's data were included in this analysis. The average number of review cycles for the incomplete cohorts may increase as those reviews are completed but will not decrease.

[g]This analysis includes only those original PMAs for which FDA or the sponsor had made a final decision; this includes reviews by CBER through September 30, 2011, and reviews by CDRH through December 1, 2011. For this analysis, the FYs 2009 through 2011 original PMA cohorts were considered still incomplete. Specifically, 22 percent of the FY 2009 original PMA cohort, 46.3 percent of the FY 2010 cohort, and 65.1 percent of the FY 2011 cohort had not yet received a final decision. As a result, it was too soon to tell what the final results for these cohorts would be. It is possible that some of the reviews taking the most time were among those not completed when we received FDA's data. The percentages of final decisions that were approval, denial, or withdrawal and the average time to final decision for original PMAs not meeting the 295-day time frame for the FYs 2009 through 2011 cohorts may increase or decrease as those reviews are completed. The average number of review cycles for the FYs 2009 through 2011 cohorts may increase as those reviews are completed but will not decrease.

[h]For the FYs 2010 through 2011 cohorts, there were no original PMAs that had received a final decision that did not meet the 295-day time frame.

Table 6: FDA Premarket Approval (PMA) Review Performance for Expedited PMAs, FYs 2000–2011

	Pre-MDUFMA			MDUFMA					MDUFA			
Fiscal years	2000	2001	2002	2003	2004	2005	2006	2007	2008	2009	2010[a]	2011[a]
Total number of submissions	11	10	12	4	17	6	3	2	4	4	6	7
Number reviewed in ≤ 180 days[b]	2	3	3	2	8	1	0	0	1	2	2	1
Percentage reviewed in ≤ 180 days[b]	18.2	30.0	25.0	50.0	47.1	16.7	0.0	0.0	25.0	50.0	40.0	50.0
Tier 1 goal percentage[c]	—	—	—	—	—	—	—	—	50	50	50	50
Met Tier 1 goal[d]	n/a	n/a	n/a	n/a	n/a	n/a	n/a	n/a	No	Yes	No[e]	Yes[e]
Number reviewed in ≤ 300 days[b]	8	6	11	3	14	5	2	0	2	3	5	2
Percentage reviewed in ≤ 300 days[b]	72.7	60.0	91.7	75.0	82.4	83.3	66.7	0.0	50.0	75.0	100.0	100.0
≤ 300 days goal percentage[c]	—	—	—	—	—	70	80	90	—	—	—	—
Met ≤ 300 days goal[d]	n/a	n/a	n/a	n/a	n/a	Yes	No	No	n/a	n/a	n/a	n/a
Number reviewed in ≤ 280 days[b]	7	6	10	3	14	4	1	0	2	3	5	2
Percentage reviewed in ≤ 280 days[b]	63.6	60.0	83.3	75.0	82.4	66.7	33.3	0.0	50.0	75.0	100.0	100.0
Tier 2 goal percentage[c]	—	—	—	—	—	—	—	—	90	90	90	90
Met Tier 2 goal[d]	n/a	n/a	n/a	n/a	n/a	n/a	n/a	n/a	No	No	Yes[e]	Yes[e]
Average number of review cycles per submission[f]	2.45	2.60	2.08	2.75	2.29	3.50	4.00	3.00	2.75	2.50	2.00	2.00
Of first-cycle decisions, percentage that were approval	0.0	20.0	16.7	0.0	17.6	16.7	0.0	0.0	25.0	0.0	16.7	14.3
Among expedited PMAs with a final decision, percentage of final decisions that were:												
Approval[g]	81.8	90.0	75.0	75.0	81.3	66.7	100.0	0.0	25.0	75.0	75.0	100.0
Denial[g]	0.0	0.0	0.0	0.0	0.0	0.0	0.0	0.0	25.0	0.0	0.0	0.0
Withdrawal[g]	18.2	10.0	25.0	25.0	18.8	33.3	0.0	100.0	50.0	25.0	25.0	0.0
Average FDA review time (in days) for expedited PMAs that were not reviewed within 280 days[b]	343	425	308	447	483	427	511	344	489	414	—[h]	—[h]
Average time to final decision (in days) for expedited PMAs that were not reviewed within 280 days[g]	588	520	334	1125	713	939	792	1111	1017	483	—[h]	—[h]

Source: GAO analysis of FDA data.

Notes: A review cohort includes all the medical device submissions relating to a particular performance goal that were submitted in a given fiscal year. For example, all expedited PMAs received by FDA from October 1, 2010, to September 30, 2011, make up the expedited PMA review cohort for FY 2011. Cohorts were considered complete if fewer than 10 percent of submissions were still under review at the time we received FDA's data. All cohorts except FY 2010 and FY 2011 were complete for the purposes of our analysis. As a result, it was too soon to tell what the final results for these cohorts would be.

We treated PMA submissions as meeting the time frame for a given performance goal if they were reviewed within the goal time plus any extension to the goal time that may have been made. The only reason the goal time can be extended is if the sponsor submits a major amendment to the submission on its own initiative (i.e., unsolicited by FDA).

[a]The FYs 2010 and 2011 expedited PMA cohorts were considered still incomplete. Specifically, 33 percent of the FY 2010 expedited PMA cohort and 71.4 percent of the FY 2011 cohort had not yet received a final decision; this includes reviews by CBER through September 30, 2011, and reviews by CDRH through December 1, 2011. Additionally, for 16.7 percent of the FY 2010 expedited PMA cohort and 71.4 percent of the FY 2011 cohort, FDA had not yet made a decision that would permanently stop the review clock for purposes of determining whether FDA met its performance goals (i.e., an approval, approvable, not approvable, withdrawal, or denial) at the time we received FDA's data. As a result, it was too soon to tell what the final results for these cohorts would be. It is possible that some of the reviews taking the most time were among those not completed when we received FDA's data. The percentage of expedited PMAs reviewed within 180 days for the FY 2010 and FY 2011 cohorts may increase or decrease as those reviews are completed; the number reviewed within 180 days and the number and percentage reviewed within 300 days and within 280 days may decrease as those reviews are completed. The percentages of final decisions that were approval, denial, or withdrawal and the average time to final decision for the FYs 2010 through 2011 cohorts may increase or decrease as those reviews are completed. The average number of review cycles for the FYs 2010 through 2011 cohorts may increase as those reviews are completed but will not decrease.

[b]Only expedited PMAs that had received a decision permanently stopping the review clock were used to determine the number and percentage of expedited PMAs reviewed within 180, 300, and 280 days.

[c]Fiscal years for which there was no corresponding expedited PMA performance goal are denoted with a dash (—).

[d]"n/a" denotes not applicable. In these years, there was no corresponding expedited PMA performance goal and therefore no determination of whether the goal was met.

[e]These results may change as the remaining expedited PMA submissions for the FY 2010 and FY 2011 cohorts receive decisions that permanently stop the review clock for purposes of determining whether FDA met its performance goals.

[f]Cycles that were currently in progress at the time we received FDA's data were included in this analysis. The average number of review cycles for the incomplete cohorts may increase as those reviews are completed but will not decrease.

[g]Only expedited PMAs that had received a final decision were used to determine the percentages of final decisions that were approval, denial, or withdrawal, and the average time to final decision for expedited PMAs not reviewed within 280 days.

[h]For the FYs 2010 through 2011 cohorts, there were no expedited PMAs that had received a final decision that did not meet the 280-day time frame.

Appendix II: Number of Full-time Equivalent (FTE) FDA Staff Supporting Medical Device User Fee Activities, FYs 2003 through 2010

FDA centers and offices	Number of FTEs in each fiscal year							
	2003	2004	2005	2006	2007	2008	2009	2010
Center for Devices and Radiological Health (CDRH)								
Office of the Center Director (OCD)[a]	13	12	15	19	34	35	52	63
Office of Management Operations (OSM/OMO)	89	62	64	62	61	50	48	52
Office of Information Technology (OIT)[b]	—	—	—	—	—	16	15	17
Office of Compliance (OC)	40	46	54	55	56	61	60	60
Office of Device Evaluation (ODE)	305	301	298	287	311	326	322	329
Office of Science and Engineering Laboratories (OST/OSEL)	88	94	110	91	89	86	87	94
Office of Communication Education and Radiation Programs (OHIP/OCER)	42	42	47	35	45	43	35	43
Office of Surveillance and Biometrics (OSB)	86	92	104	106	98	105	117	139
Office of In Vitro Diagnostics (OIVD)[c]	—	49	61	67	65	71	69	105
Committee Conference Management (CCM)[d]	—	—	—	—	—	1	1	1
CDRH Total	**662**	**697**	**753**	**721**	**760**	**793**	**805**	**902**
Center for Biologics Evaluation and Research (CBER)								
Center Director's Office, Office of Management (OM), Office of Information Management (OIM), and Office of Communication, Outreach, and Development (OCOD)	13	15	20	23	23	23	24	28
Office of Blood Research & Review	37	43	49	70	66	66	64	64
Office of Cellular, Tissue & Gene Therapies	2	2	2	2	2	5	6	6
Office of Vaccines Research & Review	1	0	0	0	1	1	1	4
Office of Therapeutics Research & Review	1	0	0	0	0	0	0	0
Office of Biostatistics & Epidemiology	1	2	2	2	2	2	4	5
Office of Compliance & Biologics Quality	5	6	9	6	8	6	4	7
CBER Total	**59**	**68**	**81**	**104**	**101**	**102**	**103**	**114**
Office of Regulatory Affairs (ORA)								
ORA Total	**59**	**60**	**62**	**64**	**64**	**62**	**57**	**69**
Office of the Commissioner (OC)								
OC Total	**77**	**70**	**77**	**78**	**90**	**74**	**84**	**86**
Shared Service (SS)[e]								
SS Total	**—**	**20**	**60**	**53**	**57**	**64**	**60**	**59**
All Centers and Offices Total	**857**	**915**	**1,034**	**1,020**	**1,071**	**1,095**	**1,109**	**1,230**

Source: GAO analysis of FDA data.

Note: All FTE rounded to the nearest whole number. FTEs for each fiscal year may not add to the fiscal year total due to rounding. One FTE represents 40 hours of work per week conducted by a federal government employee over the course of 1 year. FTEs do not include contractors and therefore provide a partial measure of staffing resources.

[a]OCD includes Medical Device Fellowship Program employees even though the Fellows were assigned to work throughout CDRH.

[b]OIT was included in the OMO FTE total prior to FY 2008.

[c]OIVD did not exist prior to FY 2004. Also, the Radiology Devices Branch was moved from ODE to OIVD between FY 2009 and FY 2010.

[d]CCM was included in the OMO FTE total prior to FY 2008.

[e]Shared Service FTE were not separated from the center FTE until FY 2004.

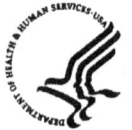

DEPARTMENT OF HEALTH & HUMAN SERVICES   OFFICE OF THE SECRETARY

Assistant Secretary for Legislation
Washington, DC 20201

FEB 22 2012

Marcia Crosse
Director, Health Care
U.S. Government Accountability Office
441 G Street NW
Washington, DC 20548

Dear Ms. Crosse:

Attached are comments on the U.S. Government Accountability Office's (GAO) report entitled, "MEDICAL DEVICES: FDA Has Met Most Performance Goals but Device Reviews Are Taking Longer" (GAO-12-418).

The Department appreciates the opportunity to review this draft section of the report prior to publication.

Sincerely,

Jim R. Esquea
Assistant Secretary for Legislation

Attachment

<u>**GENERAL COMMENTS OF THE DEPARTMENT OF HEALTH AND HUMAN
SERVICES (HHS) ON THE GOVERNMENT ACCOUNTABILITY OFFICE'S (GAO)
DRAFT REPORT ENTITLED, "MEDICAL DEVICES: FDA HAS MET MOST
PERFORMANCE GOALS BUT DEVICE REVIEWS ARE TAKING LONGER"
(GAO-12-418)**</u>

The Department appreciates the opportunity to review and comment on this draft report. As
GAO notes, the Food and Drug Administration's (FDA) own annual reports to Congress[1]
regarding medical device review times reveal the same patterns that GAO has found in this
report. FDA has continued to make progress during FY 2011 while implementing MDUFA II.
Overall, FDA has already met or exceeded, or has the potential to meet or exceed, based on
preliminary data of completed and pending reviews, 17 of 21 Tier 1 performance goals and 15 of
21 Tier 2 performance goals for the FY 2008 through FY 2011 performance goal cohorts.

In addition, GAO noted, and FDA also has identified in it own reports, that the total time to a
decision (FDA review time plus the time it takes a sponsor to provide requested information) has
increased, yet FDA's performance in meeting its goals is by and large strong. Since the total
time to a decision includes the time industry incurs in responding to FDA's concerns, FDA and
industry bear shared responsibility for the time increase and will need to work together to
improve performance on total time to decision.

FDA recently conducted an analysis of premarket review times under the 510(k) program and
identified quality issues in more than 50 percent of 510(k) applications. These quality issues
require agency staff to prepare and issue additional information letters, resulting in additional
review cycles. At the same time, FDA has been instituting management changes to improve its
premarket review programs, which the agency expects will help address the increase in total time
to decision. FDA has conducted a thorough assessment of the 510(k) review program and an
assessment of how CDRH uses science in regulatory decision-making. FDA issued two reports
in August 2010 that found that FDA needed to take several critical actions to improve the
predictability, consistency, and transparency of both the 510(k) and premarket approval
application review programs.

The agency solicited public comment on the recommendations identified in the studies and
received a range of perspectives from stakeholders, including medical device companies,
industry representatives, venture capitalists, health care professional organizations, third-party
payers, patient and consumer advocacy groups, foreign regulatory bodies, and others. After
considering the public input, in January 2011, FDA announced 25 specific actions[2] that the
agency would take to improve the predictability, consistency, and transparency of its premarket
review programs. Subsequently, FDA has taken or is taking actions to:

- create a culture change toward greater transparency, interaction, collaboration, and
  the appropriate balancing of benefits and risk;
- ensure predictable and consistent recommendations, decision-making, and application
  of the least-burdensome principle; and
- implement efficient processes and use of resources.

---

[1] http://www.fda.gov/AboutFDA/ReportsManualsForms/Reports/UserFeeReports/PerformanceReports/MDUFMA/
default.htm
[2] http://www.fda.gov/downloads/AboutFDA/CentersOffices/CDRH/CDRHReports/UCM239450.pdf

1

**GENERAL COMMENTS OF THE DEPARTMENT OF HEALTH AND HUMAN
SERVICES (HHS) ON THE GOVERNMENT ACCOUNTABILITY OFFICE'S (GAO)
DRAFT REPORT ENTITLED, "MEDICAL DEVICES: FDA HAS MET MOST
PERFORMANCE GOALS BUT DEVICE REVIEW TIMES ARE TAKING LONGER"
(GAO-12-418)**

These actions exemplify FDA's commitment to increasing the timely availability of safe and
effective new medical devices to patients and healthcare providers.

Finally, FDA needs adequate, stable funding to manage a device program that can approve or
clear safe and effective products for patients without delay, and only timely reauthorization of a
medical device user fee program that both FDA and the medical device industry support can
assure such funding.

2

Appendix IV: GAO Contact and Staff Acknowledgments

GAO Contact	Marcia Crosse, (202) 512-7114 or crossem@gao.gov:
Staff Acknowledgments	In addition to the contact named above, Robert Copeland, Assistant Director; Carolyn Fitzgerald; Cathleen Hamann; Karen Howard; Hannah Marston Minter; Lisa Motley; Aubrey Naffis; Michael Rose; and Rachel Schulman made key contributions to this report.